Atlas of Contrast-enhanced Sonography of Focal Liver Lesions

Tommaso Vincenzo Bartolotta
Adele Taibbi • Massimo Midiri

Atlas of Contrast-enhanced Sonography of Focal Liver Lesions

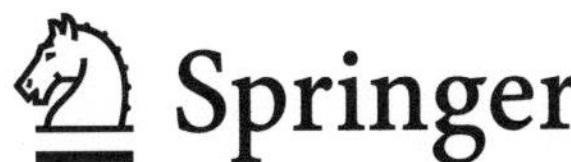

Tommaso Vincenzo Bartolotta
Department of Radiology
University Hospital
Palermo
Italy

Massimo Midiri
Department of Radiology
University Hospital
Palermo
Italy

Adele Taibbi
Department of Radiology
University Hospital
Palermo
Italy

ISBN 978-3-319-36280-9   ISBN 978-3-319-17539-3   (eBook)
DOI 10.1007/978-3-319-17539-3

Springer Cham Heidelberg New York Dordrecht London
© Springer International Publishing Switzerland 2015
Softcover reprint of the hardcover 1st edition 2015

Printed on acid-free paper

Springer International Publishing AG Switzerland is part of Springer Science+Business Media (www.springer.com)

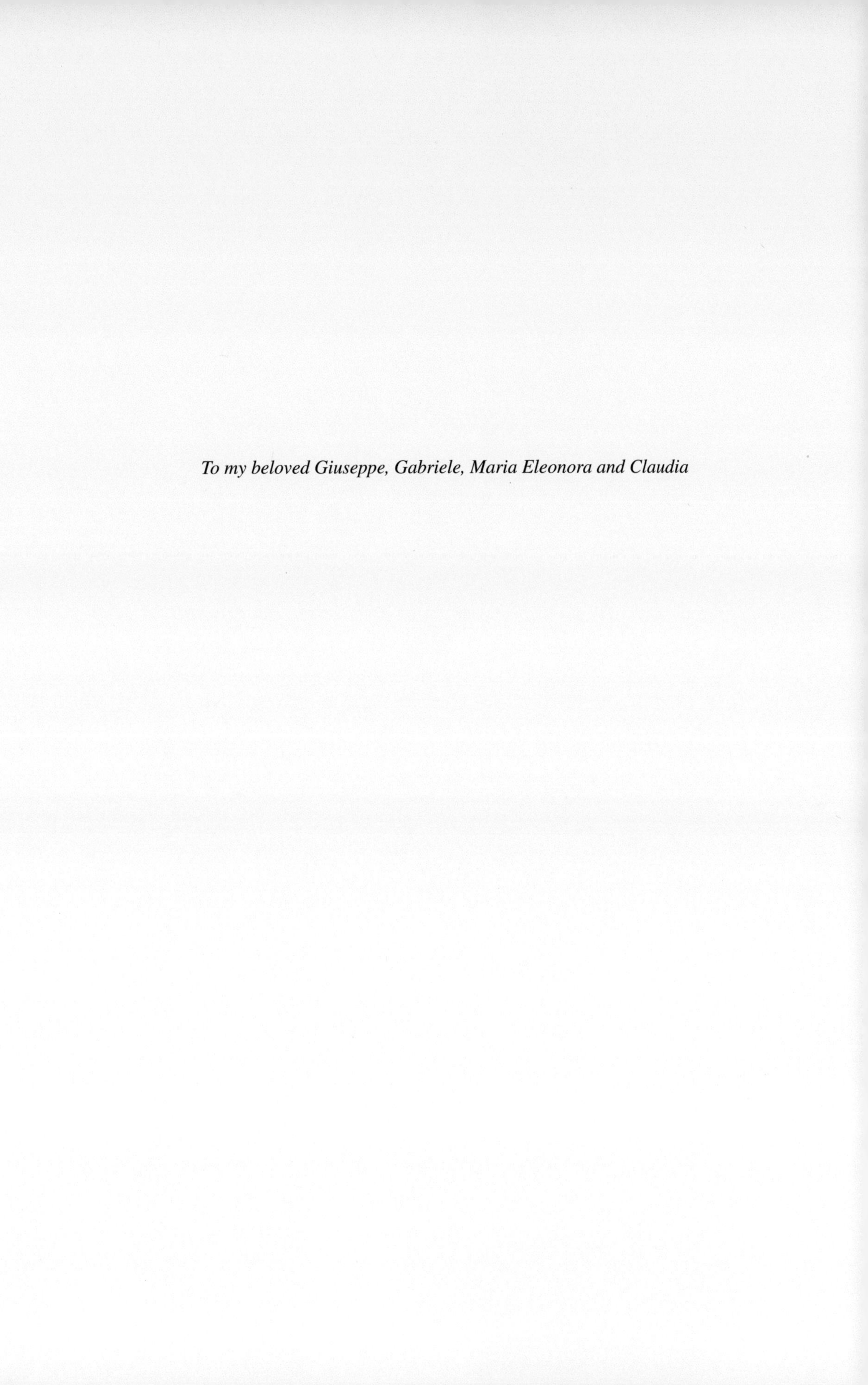

To my beloved Giuseppe, Gabriele, Maria Eleonora and Claudia

Foreword

If your pictures aren't good enough, you aren't close enough (Robert Capa)

Contrast-enhanced ultrasound (CEUS) represents a significant breakthrough in sonography and is being increasingly used for evaluation of focal liver lesions (FLLs). The unique feature of CEUS of non-invasively assessing in real time liver perfusion throughout the vascular phase has led to a dramatic improvement in diagnostic accuracy of US in either detection or characterization of FLLs, as well as in the guidance and evaluation of response of therapeutic procedures. Currently, CEUS is included in many international guidelines as a part of the suggested diagnostic workup of FLLs, resulting in a better patient management and cost-effective therapy delivery. This book offers an image-based, comprehensive quick reference guide that will assist in the interpretation of CEUS examinations of the liver in daily practice. The *Atlas of Contrast-Enhanced Sonography of Focal Liver Lesions* will serve as an invaluable hands-on tool for practitioners who need to diagnose liver lesions using CEUS in the major clinical settings: oncology patients, cirrhotic patients, and patients with incidental focal liver lesions. This book is based on the daily practice of all the authors who would like to share their endless enthusiasm and strong commitment to ultrasonography with all the colleagues who are interested in the exciting field of contrast-enhanced ultrasound of the liver.

Roberto Lagalla
Rector of the University of Palermo
Palermo, Italy

Contents

Introduction

1

1.1 General Overview

Thanks to the most recent technological innovations, the ability of grayscale ultrasound (US) in the detection of focal liver lesions (FLLs) has significantly improved, even if small or deeply located. However, the characterization remains a challenge even for experienced sonographers except for hemangiomas with typical US appearance detected in patients with no history of malignancy or chronic liver disease [1].

Both benign and malignant FLLs can present similar aspect at US, thus making really difficult a correct differential diagnosis especially when liver echotexture is altered such as in chronic hepatitis or diffuse fatty infiltration. In particular, this latter, increasing the ultrasound beam attenuation, also hinders lesion's identification, and the majority of liver masses appear hypoechoic regardless of tumor's nature.

Moreover, color and power Doppler evaluation slightly improves diagnostic performance of US examination since they visualize large vessels and are limited by motion artifacts, making the analysis often unsatisfactory and thus inconclusive for the differential diagnosis of FLLs.

In the last decades, the development of both second-generation ultrasound contrast media and specific software for contrast agent detection has significantly improved diagnostic accuracy of US in terms of sensitivity and specificity. Nowadays, contrast-enhanced ultrasound (CEUS) represents a reliable, safe, and cost-saving alternative imaging modality able to provide in most cases, in the same US session, a correct characterization of an indeterminate FLL with diagnostic accuracy comparable to CT or MR performed with state-of-the-art scanners thus significantly reducing the number of cases requiring further investigations [2, 3].

CEUS is a real-time technique thus allowing to continuously study microvessels of FLLs adding, with respect to CT and MR examinations (sometimes inconclusive), further useful information that makes it a helpful problem-solving imaging modality.

The European Federation of Societies for Ultrasound in Medicine and Biology (EFSUMB) also recommends CEUS especially in peculiar clinical settings as, for example, in the diagnosis of incidentally discovered FLLs indeterminate at US or in the evaluation of locoregional treatment.

At this regard, a newly developed CEUS technique, three-dimensional CEUS (3D-CEUS) performed by means of a 3D probe, has been reported to improve the study of tumor vascularity in the three orthogonal planes, allowing the visualization of the region of interest from different points of view.

In some cases regarding locoregional treatment CEUS evaluation, an example of a particular 3D reconstruction software called "i-slice" will be showed in this atlas. I-slice provides the

© Springer International Publishing Switzerland 2015
T.V. Bartolotta et al., *Atlas of Contrast-enhanced Sonography of Focal Liver Lesions*,
DOI 10.1007/978-3-319-17539-3_1

capability of displaying the data set in multiple, contiguous, parallel 2D slices, similar to CT and MR, changing the interval (distance between the individual slices) and the depth setting (the position of the slices in the volume) in order to better display the region of interest [4, 5].

So the aim of this atlas is to describe by means of a wide collection of clinical cases the most common imaging patterns of benign and malignant FLLs evaluated by means of CEUS in order to make the specialist who would like to perform it confident in the interpretation of imaging findings and able to provide pivotal information for a definitive characterization during the same session of a baseline US examination avoiding further imaging workup.

1.2   Physical Basis and Specific Contrast Enhancement Technique

The ultrasound contrast agents (UCAs) currently used in diagnostic US are characterized by a microbubble structure consisting of gas bubbles stabilized by a shell. UCAs act as blood pool agents. They strongly increase the US backscatter and therefore are useful in the enhancement of blood echogenicity for the assessment of blood flow in the micro- and macrovessels. SonoVue© contains low-solubility gas (sulfur hexafluoride) microbubbles surrounded by a flexible phospholipid shell improving microbubble stability. The microbubbles have a mean size of 2.5 μm with 99 % of them smaller than 11 μm allowing a free passage in the capillaries but keeping the contrast medium within the lumen.

The assessment of microbubbles usually requires contrast-specific imaging modes.

Contrast-specific US softwares are generally based on the cancellation and/or separation of linear US signals from tissue and utilization of the nonlinear response from microbubbles.

Nonlinear response from second-generation contrast agents is based on nonlinear response from microbubble oscillations at low acoustic pressure, reducing disruption of the microbubbles.

Due to the flexibility of the microbubbles' phospholipid shell, the reflectivity of SonoVue is very high with high echo enhancement. On the other hand, due to the poor solubility and diffusivity, this contrast agent is also strongly resistant to pressure. This allows minimally disruptive contrast-specific imaging at mechanical index (MI) set in clinical practice and enables effective investigations over several minutes with the visualization of the dynamic enhancement pattern in real time. Low-MI techniques furthermore lead to effective tissue signal suppression as the nonlinear response from the tissue is minimal when low acoustic pressures are used.

In summary, low-MI imaging with second-generation contrast agent (i.e., SonoVue) allows real-time examination and the evaluation of contrast medium distribution from the beginning of intravenous injection up to 4–5 min.

1.3   Technical Examination

In our department, CEUS examination involves the use of US scanners equipped with convex probe and Pulse Inversion Harmonic Imaging software, extremely sensitive to microbubble-based US contrast agents. The first part of the study includes a preliminary assessment of hepatic parenchyma in grayscale—including color power Doppler and pulsed Doppler analysis—in order to localize the lesion and select an appropriate scanning plane. Once set, the US scan parameters—such as focal zone, time gain compensation, MI—remain unchanged throughout the study. The US contrast agent (USCA) is sulfur hexafluoride filled microbubble based (SonoVue®, Bracco, Milan, Italy), intravenously injected as a 2.4 mL bolus followed by 10 mL of sterile saline flush by using a 20- or 22-gauge peripheral cannula. In order to minimize microbubble disruption, a low frame rate (5 Hz) and a low MI, usually 0.06, are used for real-time imaging.

Digital cineloops are registered, respectively, during the arterial, (i.e., 10–40 s from beginning of contrast agent bolus injection) and extended portal venous phase (i.e., until 200–300 s from beginning of injection).

Considering that currently used USCAs are blood pool agents, without any interstitial or equilibrium phase, some authors describe a unique extended portal venous phase starting just after the arterial phase and progressively fading up to 3 min [6].

All images and cineloops are digitally stored both as raw data in a PC-based workstation connected to the US units via a standard Ethernet link and sent to a Picture Archiving and Communication System (PACS).

When multiple lesions are present in the same patient, multiple doses can be injected in order to study each one with an interval time of at least 10 min making sure there are no more contrast medium microbubbles within the vessels. Otherwise, before any further injection, the entire liver parenchyma can be scanned at high MI (1.3) in order to destroy any remaining ones.

Baseline echogenicity and dynamic enhancement pattern of each lesion are evaluated in the arterial and extended portal-venous phase in comparison with adjacent liver parenchyma.

1.4 Safety

In general, UCAs are extremely safe with a low incidence of side effects. They are not nephrotoxic or cardiotoxic, and the incidence of hypersensitivity or allergic events appears much lower than current CT or MR contrast agents. It is not necessary to perform laboratory tests of renal function before administering them.

Life-threatening anaphylactoid reactions in abdominal applications have been reported with a rate of 0.001 %, with no deaths in a series of >23,000 patients [7].

Nonetheless, investigators should be trained in resuscitation and have the appropriate facilities available.

Although there is a theoretical possibility that the interaction of diagnostic ultrasound and UCA could produce bioeffects, there is no clinical evidence for adverse effects on the human liver. Cellular effects that have been observed in vitro include sonoporation, hemolysis, and cell death. Data from small animal models suggest that microvascular disruption can occur when microbubbles are insonated [8]. Thus, in general, low MI should be preferred for CEUS of the liver. Some general recommendations include the following: (a) as in all diagnostic ultrasound procedures, the operator should be mindful of the desirability of keeping the displayed MI low and of avoiding unduly long exposure times; (b) caution should be exercised when using UCA in patients with severe coronary artery disease, clinically unstable ischemic cardiac disease, right-to-left shunts, severe pulmonary hypertension, uncontrolled systemic hypertension, and adult respiratory distress syndrome; (c) as with all contrast agents, resuscitation facilities must be available; (d) the use of UCA should be avoided 24 h prior to extracorporeal shock wave therapy [9].

Caution with respect to the use of UCAs in these cardiac instances derives from an anecdotal temporal but unproven causal association between contrast injection and death in severely compromised cardiac patients. However, in very large patient cohorts, the use of UCAs for acute cardiac patients has been shown to be associated with a decreased, not increased, risk of death thanks to the efficacy of the modality [10, 11].

UCAs are not licensed in pregnancy or in pediatric patients. Nevertheless, some authors have recently reported their experience about off-label use of UCA in pediatric patients [12, 13].

References

1. Bartolotta TV, Taibbi A, Midiri M, Matranga D, Solbiati L, Lagalla R (2011) Indeterminate focal liver lesions incidentally discovered at gray-scale US: role of contrast-enhanced sonography. Invest Radiol 46(2):106–115
2. Malhi H, Grant EG, Duddalwar V (2014) Contrast-enhanced ultrasound of the liver and kidney. Radiol Clin North Am 52(6):1177–1190
3. Cantisani V, Grazhdani H, Fioravanti C, Rosignuolo M, Calliada F, Messineo D, Bernieri MG, Redler A, Catalano C, D'Ambrosio F (2014) Liver metastases: contrast-enhanced ultrasound compared with computed tomography and magnetic resonance. World J Gastroenterol 20(29):9998–10007
4. Bartolotta TV, Taibbi A, Midiri M, De Maria M (2008) Hepatocellular cancer response to radiofre-

quency tumor ablation: contrast-enhanced ultrasound. Abdom Imaging 33(5):501–511

5. Bartolotta TV, Taibbi A, Matranga D, Midiri M, Lagalla R (2015) 3D versus 2D contrast-enhanced sonography in the evaluation of therapeutic response of hepatocellular carcinoma after locoregional therapies: preliminary findings. Radiol Med [Epub ahead of print]

6. Burns PN, Wilson SR (2007) Focal liver masses: enhancement patterns on contrast-enhanced images—concordance of US scans with CT scans and MR images. Radiology 242:162–174

7. Piscaglia F, Bolondi L, Italian Society for Ultrasound in Medicine and Biology (SIUMB) Study Group on Ultrasound Contrast Agents (2006) The safety of Sonovue in abdominal applications: retrospective analysis of 23188 investigations. Ultrasound Med Biol 32(9):1369–1375

8. Skyba DM, Price RJ, Linka AZ, Skalak TC, Kaul S (1998) Direct in vivo visualization of intravascular destruction of microbubbles by ultrasound and its local effects on tissue. Circulation 98(4):290–293

9. Claudon M, Dietrich CF, Choi BI, Cosgrove DO, Kudo M, Nolsøe CP, Piscaglia F, Wilson SR, Barr RG, Chammas MC, Chaubal NG, Chen M-H, Clevert DA, Correas JM, Ding H, Forsberg F, Fowlkes JB, Gibson RN, Goldberg BB, Lassau N, Leen ELS, Mattrey RF, Moriyasu F, Solbiati L, Weskott H-P, Xu H-X (2013) Guidelines and good clinical practice recommendations for Contrast Enhanced Ultrasound (CEUS) in the liver – update 2012. A WFUMB-EFSUMB initiative in cooperation with representatives of AFSUMB, AIUM, ASUM, FLAUS and ICUS. Ultrasound Med Biol 39(2):187–210

10. Main ML, Goldman JH, Grayburn PA (2009) Ultrasound contrast agents: balancing safety versus efficacy. Expert Opin Drug Saf 8:49–56

11. Main ML, Ryan AC, Davis TE et al (2008) Acute mortality in hospitalized patients undergoing echocardiography with and without an ultrasound contrast agent (multicenter registry results in 4,300,966 consecutive patients). Am J Cardiol 102:1742–1746

12. Coleman JL, Navid F, Furman WL, McCarville MB (2014) Safety of ultrasound contrast agents in the pediatric oncologic population: a single-institution experience. AJR Am J Roentgenol 202(5):966–970

13. Schreiber-Dietrich DG, Cui XW, Piscaglia F, Gilja OH, Dietrich CF (2014) Contrast enhanced ultrasound in pediatric patients: a real challenge. Z Gastroenterol 52(10):1178–1184

Benign Focal Liver Lesions

2.1 Hepatic Cysts

A simple hepatic cyst is a single, unilocular lesion containing homogeneous serous fluid surrounded by a single layer of cuboidal epithelium, identical to that of bile ducts, and a thin underlying layer of fibrous stroma [1].

Usually, a correct diagnosis is already allowed by means of grayscale US thanks to a homogeneous anechoic appearance, a thin or imperceptible wall with posterior acoustic enhancement. Some internal thin septa may be present, but thick septa should suggest an abscess, parasitic infection, or cystic neoplasm. In particular, at CEUS, cystic tumors of biliary origin and cystic metastasis usually present a thick capsule, thick internal septa, or mural nodules which show contrast enhancement suggesting the presence of viable tissue [2].

Furthermore, hemorrhagic or complicated cysts may show hypoechoic inhomogeneous appearance instead of typical anechoic aspect on conventional US scan. In these cases, CEUS can depict the absence of vascularization throughout the vascular phase, suggesting cystic nature.

© Springer International Publishing Switzerland 2015
T.V. Bartolotta et al., *Atlas of Contrast-enhanced Sonography of Focal Liver Lesions*,
DOI 10.1007/978-3-319-17539-3_2

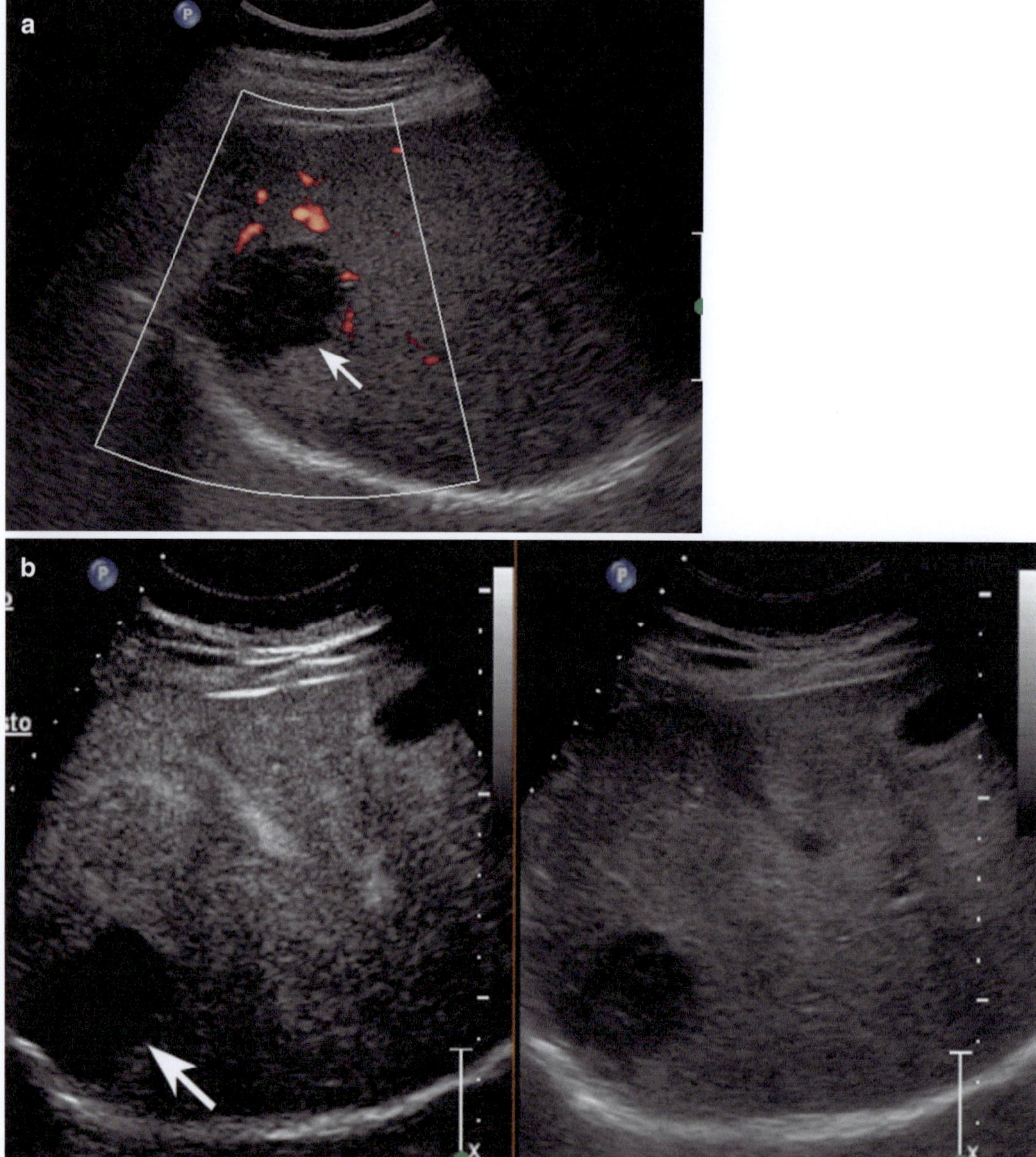

Fig. 2.1 Complicated cyst in a 48-year-old man. (**a**) Oblique ascending right subcostal baseline image shows a markedly hypoechoic lesion sized 3.5 cm in the subcapsular region of the VII hepatic segment not showing vascu-lar signal at power-Doppler evaluation (*arrow*). (**b–d**) At CEUS, the lesion shows lack of contrast enhancement throughout the vascular phases (*arrows*)

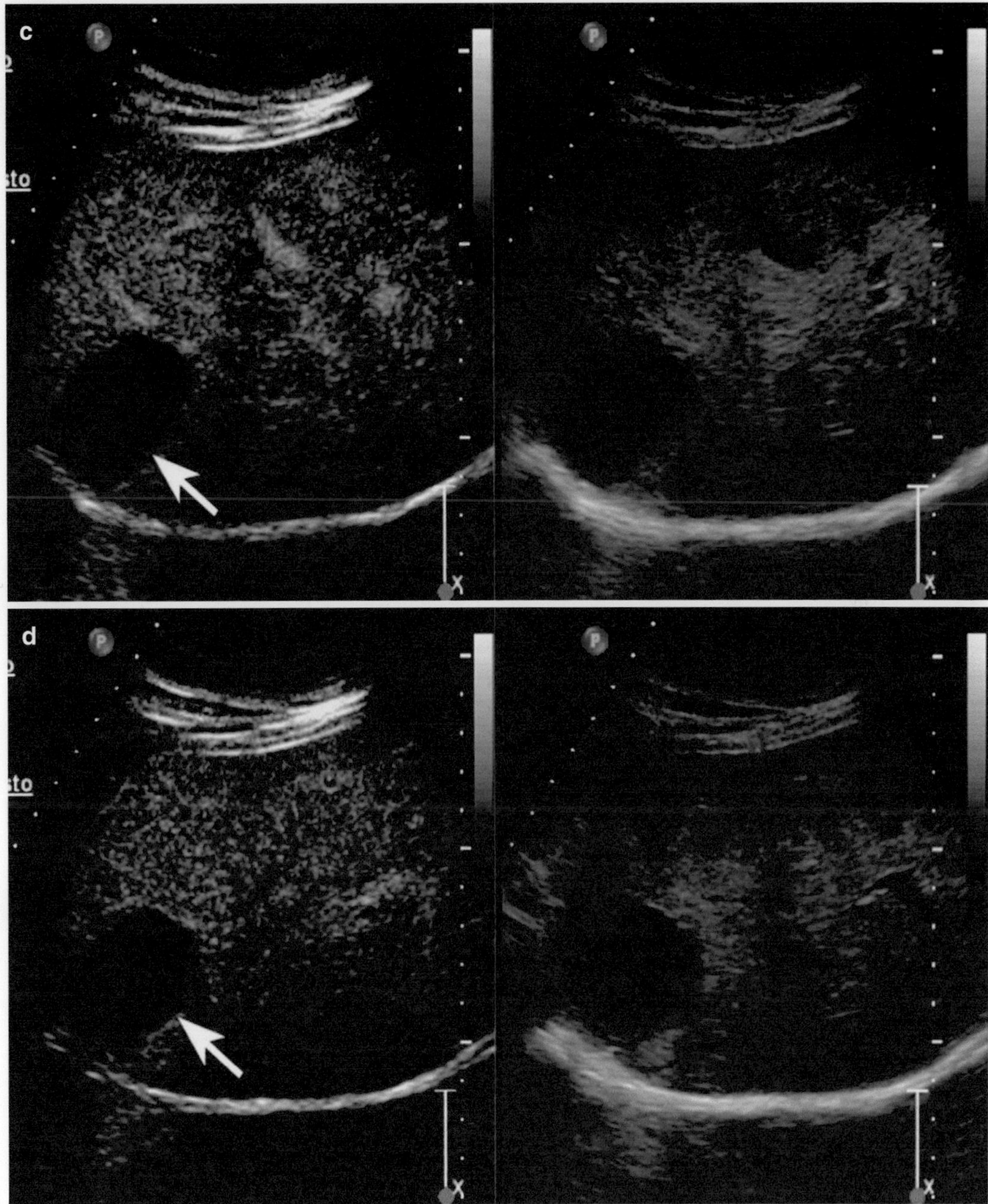

Fig. 2.1 (continued)

2.2 Hydatid Cyst

Hydatid disease is a parasitic infestation by a tapeworm of the genus Echinococcus.

Cystic hydatid disease usually affects the liver (50–70 %) and less frequently the lung, the spleen, the kidney, the bones, and the brain. Liver hydatidosis can cause dissemination or anaphylaxis after a cyst ruptures into the peritoneum or biliary tract. Infection of the cyst can facilitate the development of liver abscesses and mechanic local complications, such as mass effect on bile ducts and vessels that can induce cholestasis, portal hypertension, and Budd-Chiari syndrome. At baseline US, hydatid cysts may present a solid aspect because of its inhomogeneous complex appearance. Parasitic cyst usually presents as a single, unilocular cyst or multiseptated cysts, showing "wheel-like," "rosette-like," or "honeycomb-like" appearances. "Snowstorm" sign may appear as multiple internal echogenic foci within the cyst cavity (hydatid sand). A correct diagnosis is of clinical relevance since biopsy of these lesions is not recommended in order to avoid severe adverse events. Usually, CEUS shows lack of enhancement of septa separating daughter cysts [3, 4].

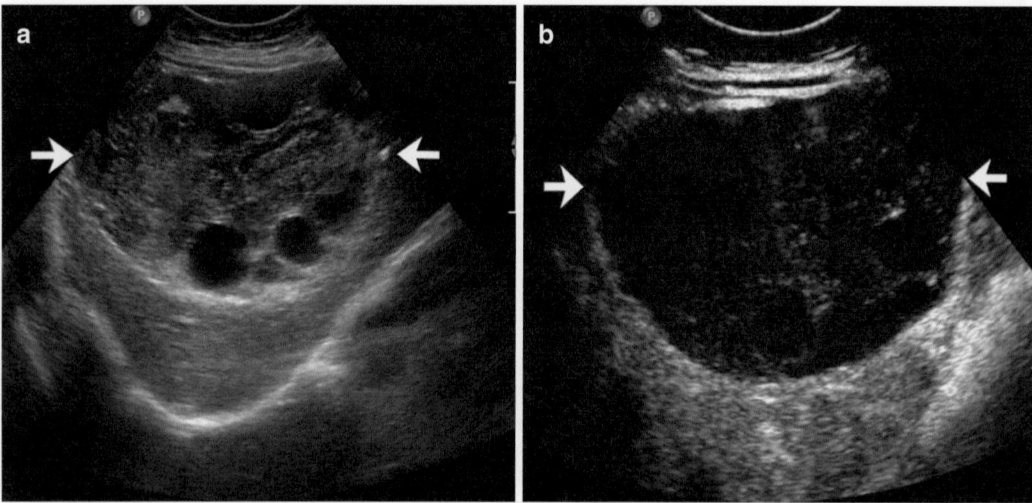

Fig. 2.2 Hydatid cyst with daughter cysts in a 62-year-old man. (**a**) At baseline US, a large heterogeneous hypoechoic mass sized 13.1 cm with multiple internal cystic areas is detected in the right hepatic lobe (*arrows*). (**b**) CEUS depicts the lesion as a constantly avascular mass (*arrows*)

2.3 Hemangioma

Hemangioma is the most frequent primary benign tumor of the liver found out with a prevalence range varying from 1 to 20 % and a higher incidence in females (women/men: 2/1–5/1).

At histopathological analysis, hemangioma is characterized by vascular lacunae lined by a single layer of endothelial cells associated with a variable rate of fibrous tissue [5, 6]. The differential diagnosis with other hepatic lesions has a pivotal clinical impact since it does not require any treatment.

At grayscale US, the hemangioma can present a "typical" aspect—hyperechoic lesion, variable in size with homogeneous or slightly inhomogeneous echotexture, well-defined margins with or without posterior wall shadowing—making easy a correct diagnosis especially in patients with no history of malignancy or chronic liver disease. Usually, color- and power-Doppler evaluation does not show any vascular signal within or at the periphery of the lesion because of very slow blood flows that distinguish it. Except for patients with cancer history or known chronic HBV-HCV-related liver disease, the detection of a lesion presenting these imaging findings does not require any further investigation.

Nevertheless, on grayscale US, hemangioma may show atypical features, such as an inhomogeneous internal echotexture. In particular, hemangiomas larger than 4–5 cm may present a markedly inhomogeneous aspect, because of thrombohemorrhagic episodes, cystic degeneration, fibrosis or hyalinization, and calcium deposit [7]. In these latter cases, CEUS represents a useful tool in order to more precisely characterize the lesion demonstrating, as shown at contrast-enhanced CT and MR, peculiar and specific contrast enhancement patterns [8–10]. In fact, CEUS allows the depiction of typical peripheral nodular enhancement in the arterial phase followed by a progressive centripetal fill-in in the extended portal-venous phase, which is considered diagnostic for hemangioma on contrast-enhanced CT and MR [11]. Incomplete fill-in in the extended portal-venous phase can depend either on the lesion size and the presence of thrombohemorrhagic phenomena or fibrosis [12]. In a smaller percentage of cases, it is possible to observe a peripheral rim enhancement in the arterial phase followed by a progressive centripetal complete or incomplete fill-in [13]. And finally, lesions smaller than 2 cm can show a rapid and homogeneous uptake of contrast medium in the arterial phase with sustained contrast enhancement in the remaining phases [14]. This feature is suggestive of capillary hemangioma. Capillary hemangioma could cause misinterpretation since other benign (focal nodular hyperplasia, hepatocellular adenoma) and malignant lesions (well-differentiated hepatocellular carcinoma) present this contrast enhancement behavior. Hence, clinical history is of pivotal relevance since if a lesion presenting these findings at CEUS is found out in a patient with chronic hepatitis, further investigations such as MR with hepatocellular-specific contrast medium are needed in order to rule out a well-differentiated hepatocellular carcinoma or a dysplastic nodule [15, 16].

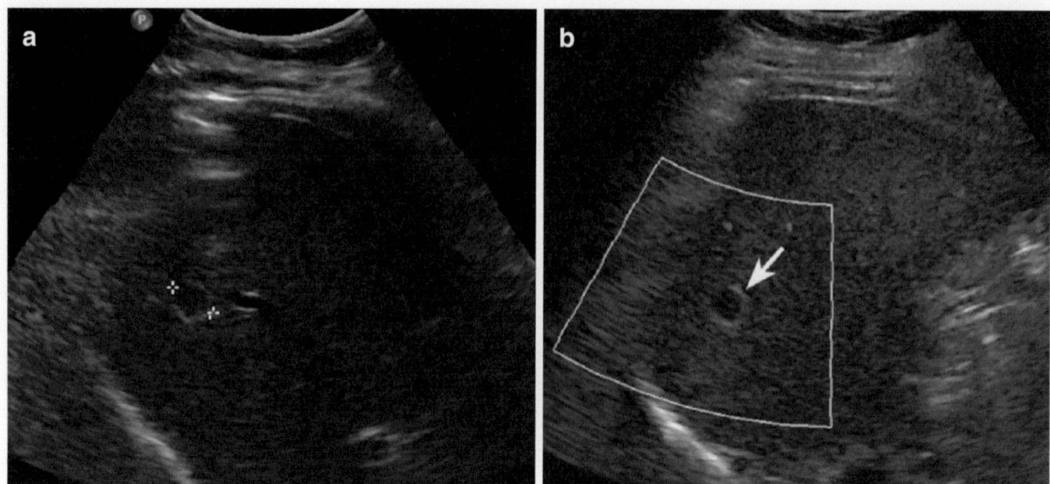

Fig. 2.3 Capillary hemangioma. (**a**) Baseline image shows an inhomogeneous lesion with hypoechoic central area surrounded by peripheral hyperechoic rim, sized 1.2 cm in the VII-VIII hepatic segment in a 52-years-old woman (*calipers*). (**b**) No vascular signal is evident at color-Doppler evaluation (*arrow*). (**c**) At CEUS in the arterial phase, the lesion presents a rapid and homogeneous uptake of contrast agent (*arrow*). The lesion is isovascular to the surrounding liver parenchyma in the late phase (**d**)

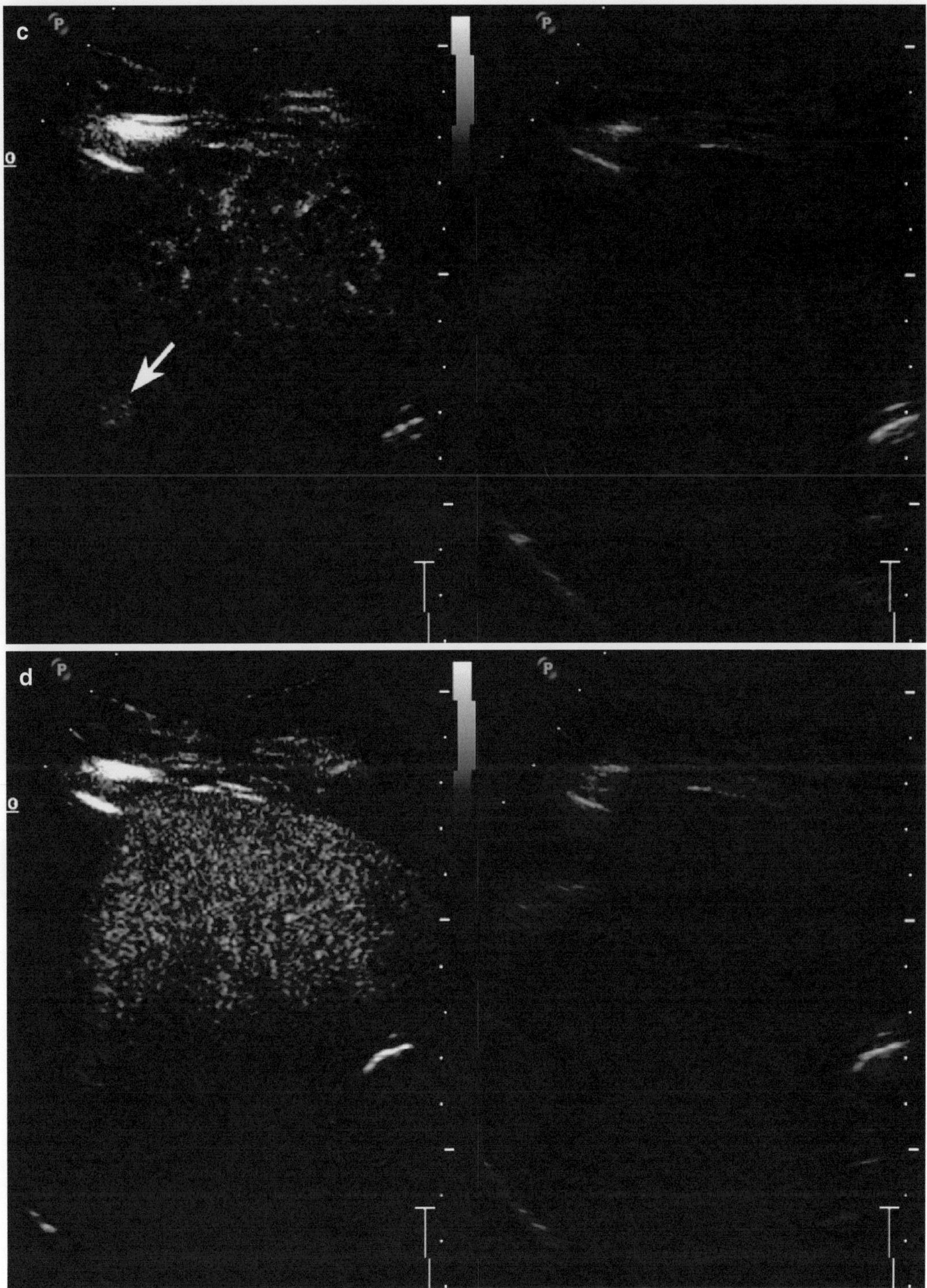

Fig. 2.3 (continued)

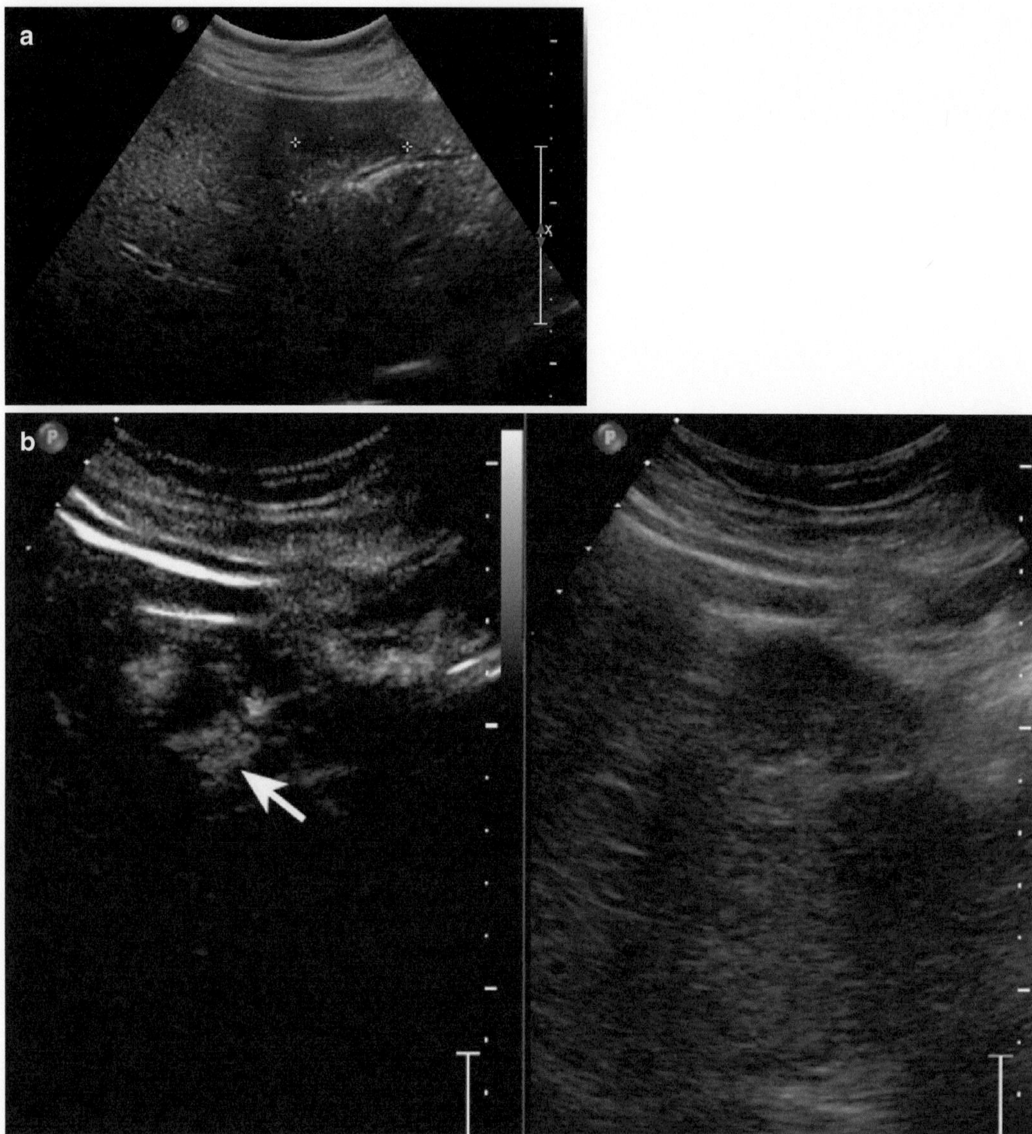

Fig. 2.4 Hemangioma in a 58-year-old man. (**a**) Baseline US image shows an homogeneous hypoechoic 3.6 cm-sized lesion, located in segment IV in the subcapsular region (*calipers*). (**b**) At CEUS, globular peripheral enhancement is appreciable in the arterial phase (*arrow*), followed by a progressive complete centripetal fill-in in the portal-venous phase (**c**). (**d**) The lesion is isoechoic with respect to the surrounding liver parenchyma in the late phase (*arrow*)

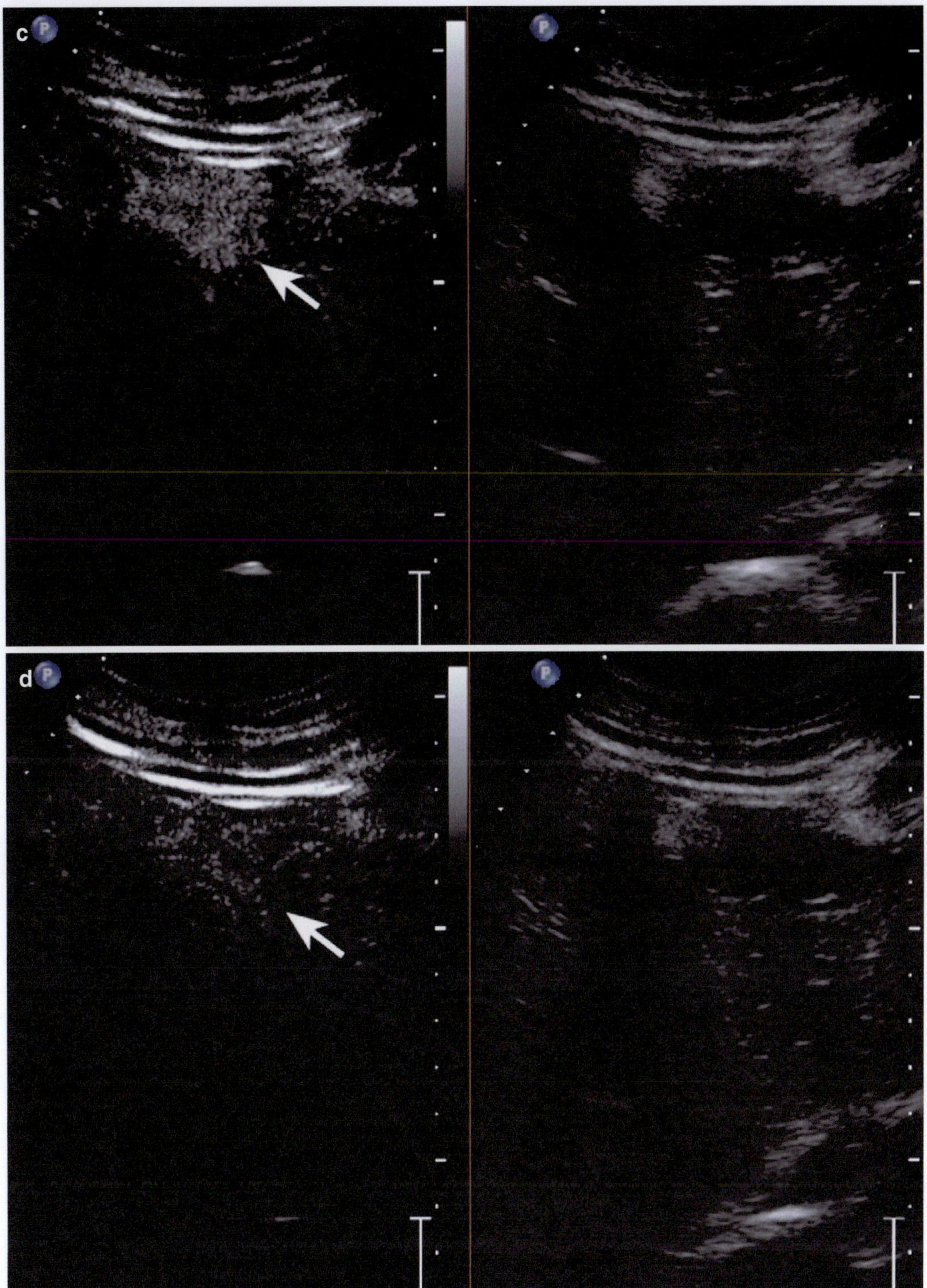

Fig. 2.4 (continued)

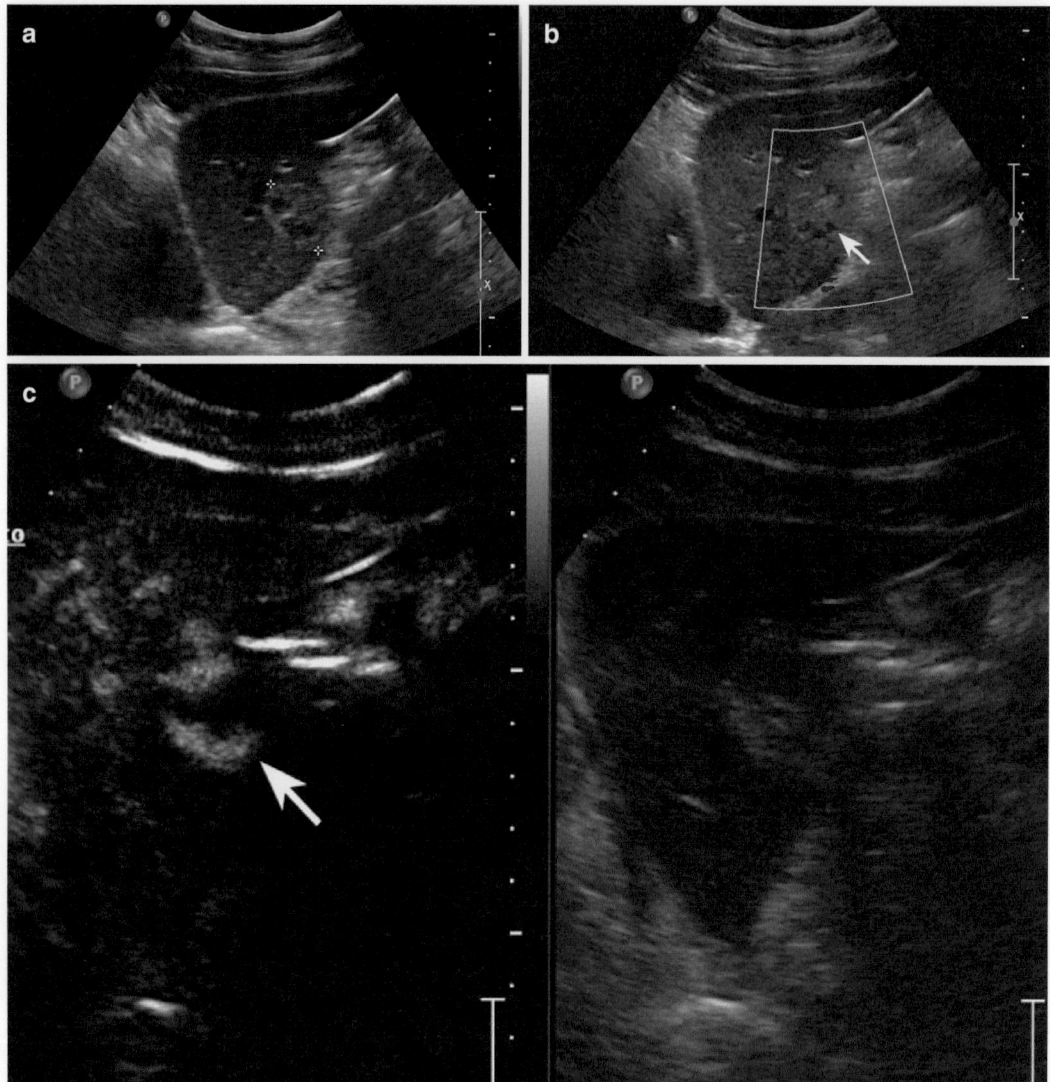

Fig. 2.5 Haemangioma in a 65-year-old woman. (**a**) Baseline US image shows a moderately inhomogeneous hyperechoic lesion, 2.9 cm in size, located in segment III in the subcapsular region (*calipers*). (**b**) No vascular signal is evident at color-Doppler evaluation (*arrow*). (**c**) At CEUS, globular peripheral enhancement is appreciable in the arterial phase (*arrow*), followed by a progressive centripetal fill-in in the portal-venous phase (**d**), incomplete in the late phase (**e**) (*arrows*)

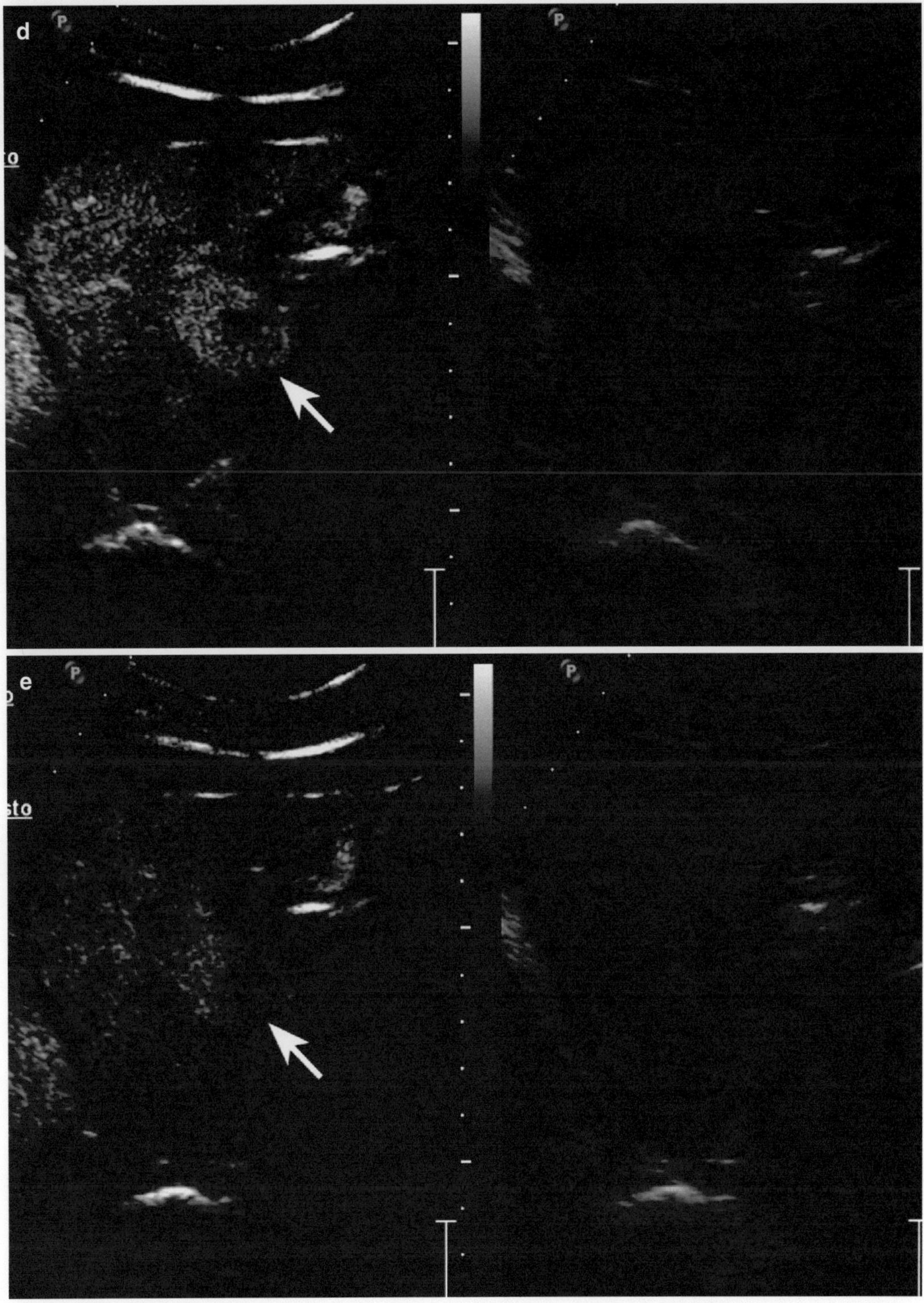

Fig. 2.5 (continued)

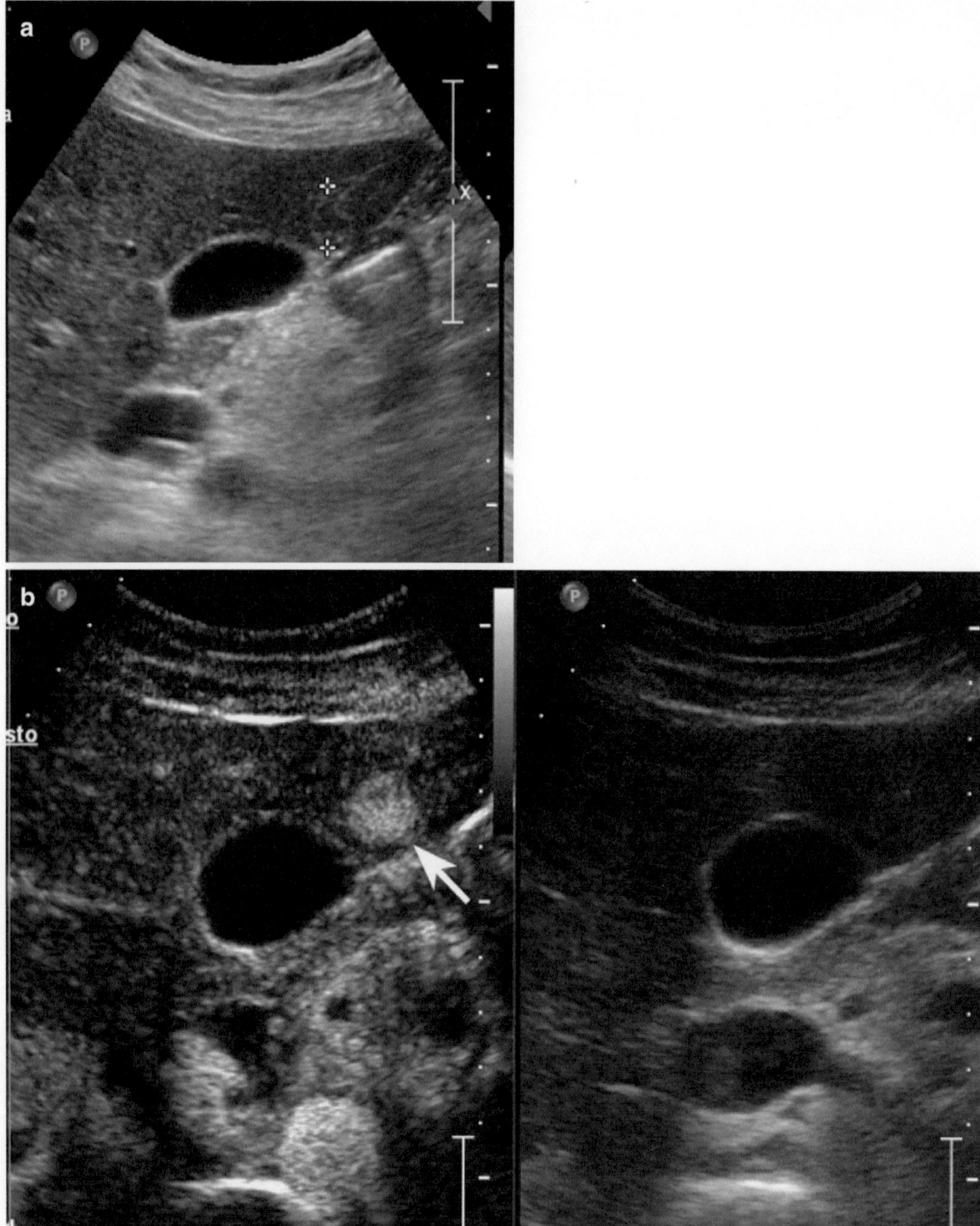

Fig. 2.6 Capillary hemangioma in a 45-year-old man. (**a**) Baseline image shows an inhomogeneous moderately hyperechoic lesion sized 1.4 cm in the IV hepatic segment (*calipers*). (**b**) At CEUS in the arterial phase, the lesion shows a rapid and homogeneous uptake of contrast agent (*arrow*). The lesion reveals a sustained contrast enhancement remaining hyperechoic with respect to the surrounding liver parenchyma during the portal-venous (**c**) and late phases (**d**) (*arrows*)

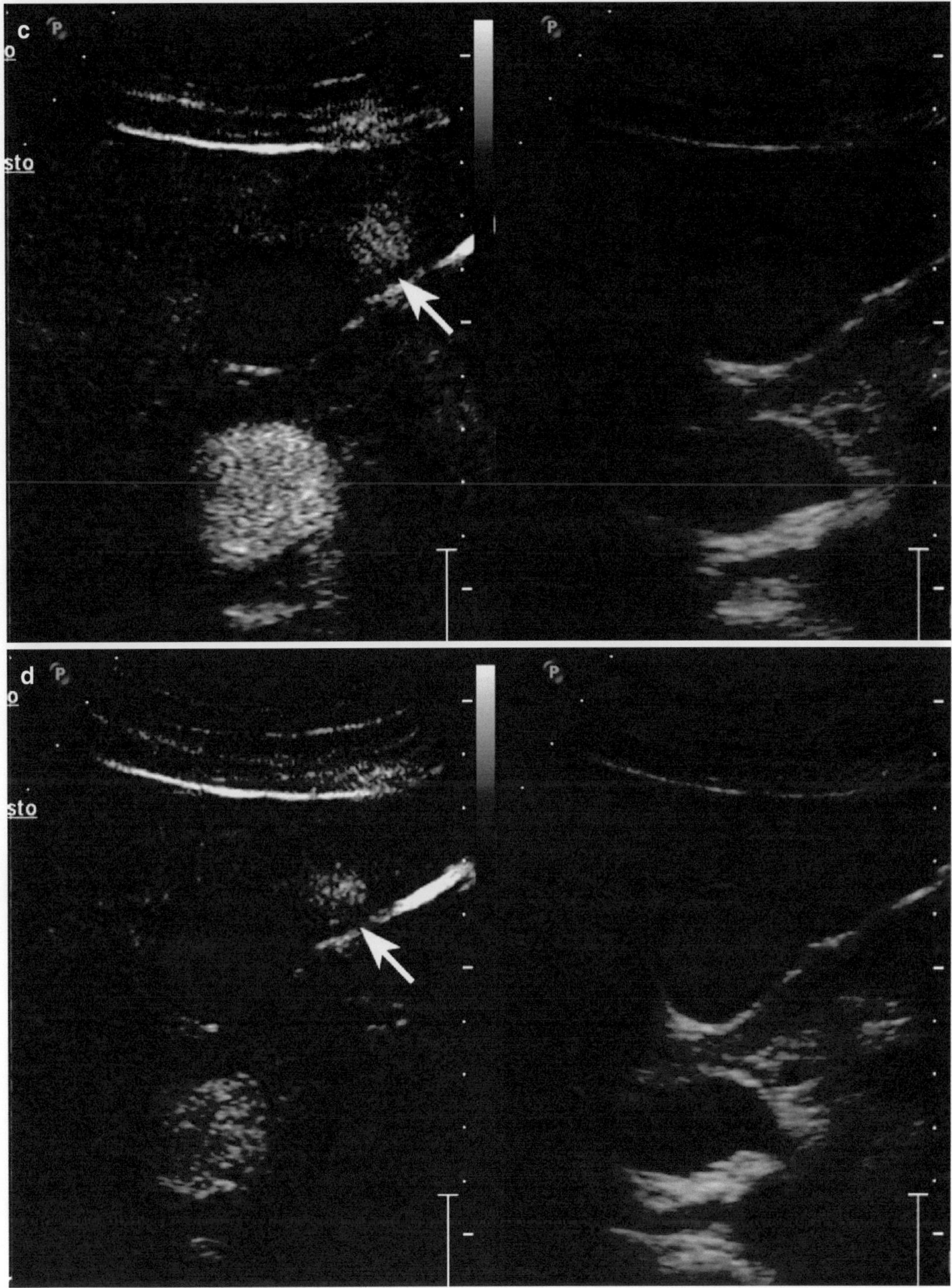

Fig. 2.6 (continued)

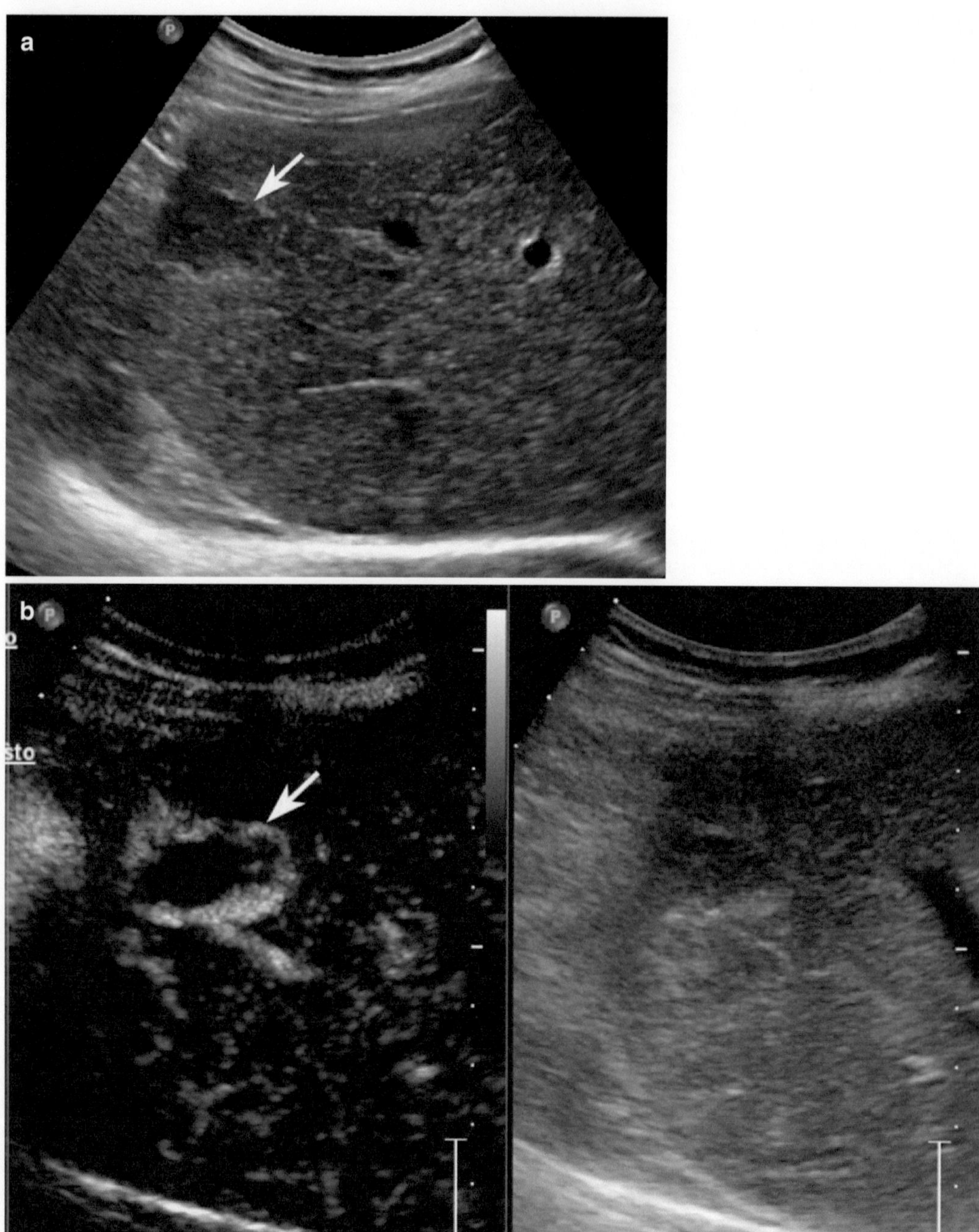

Fig. 2.7 Hemangioma in a 54-year-old asymptomatic woman. (**a**) Baseline US shows a slightly hypoechoic homogeneous lesion, 2.2 cm in size, located in segment VI in the subcapsular region (*arrow*). (**b**) At CEUS, globular peripheral enhancement is appreciable in the arterial phase (*arrow*), followed by a progressive centripetal fill-in, complete in the remaining vascular phases (**c, d**) (*arrows*). (**e**) 3D i-Slice reconstruction shows globular peripheral enhancement in each slice too

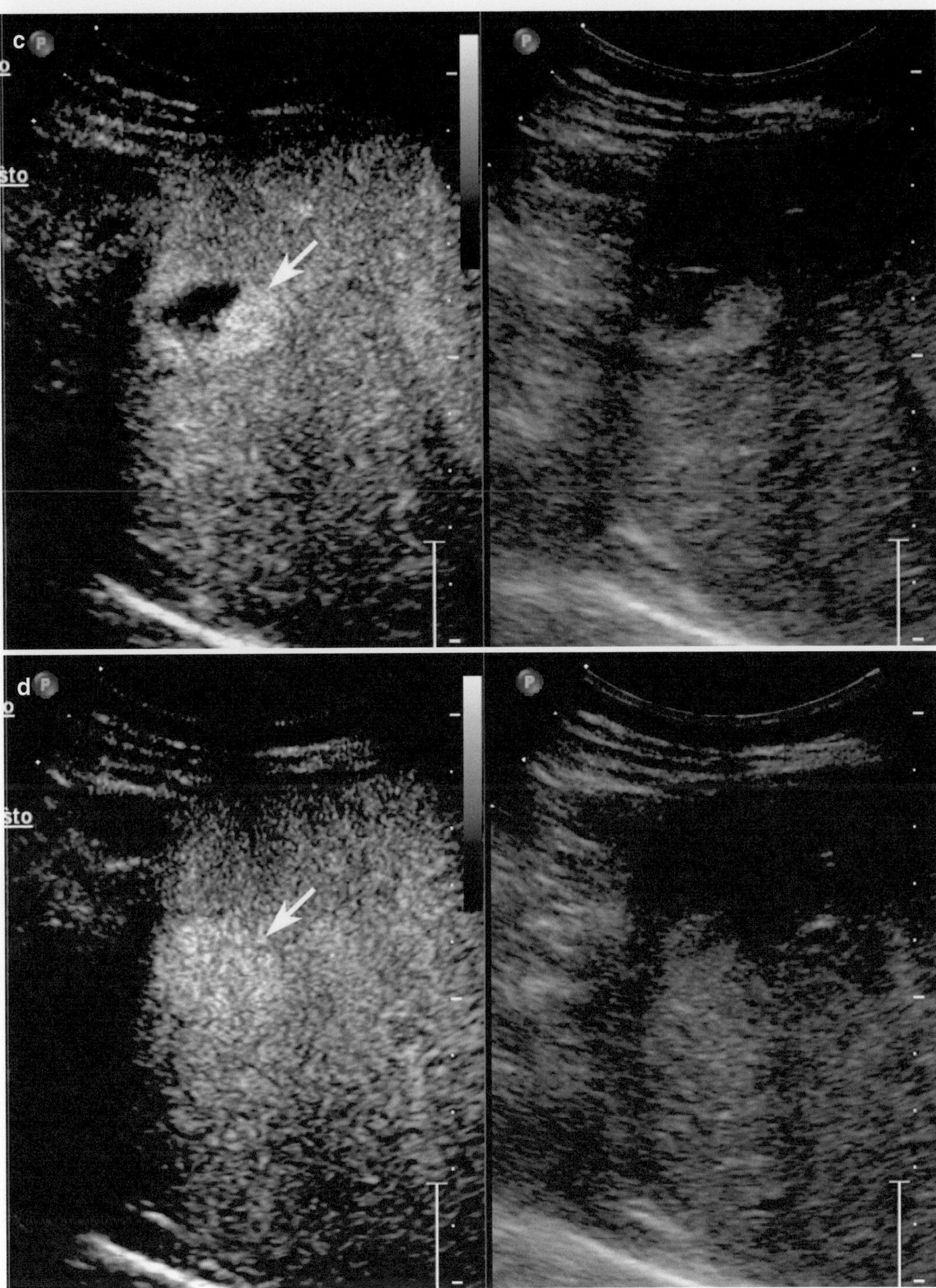

Fig. 2.7 (continued)

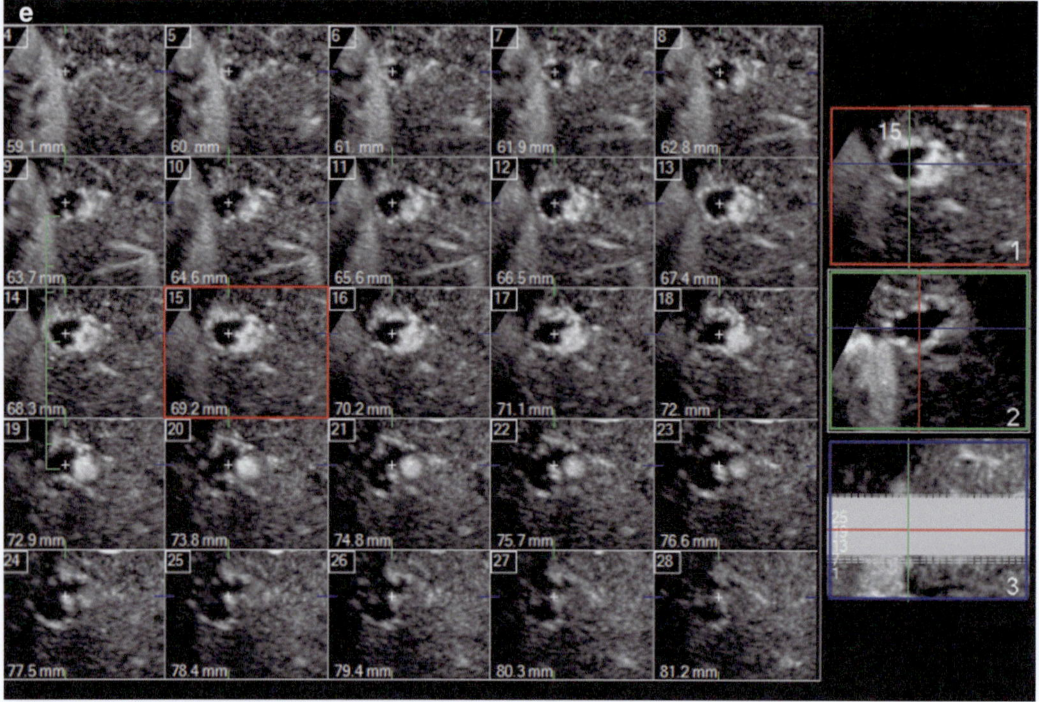

Fig. 2.7 (continued)

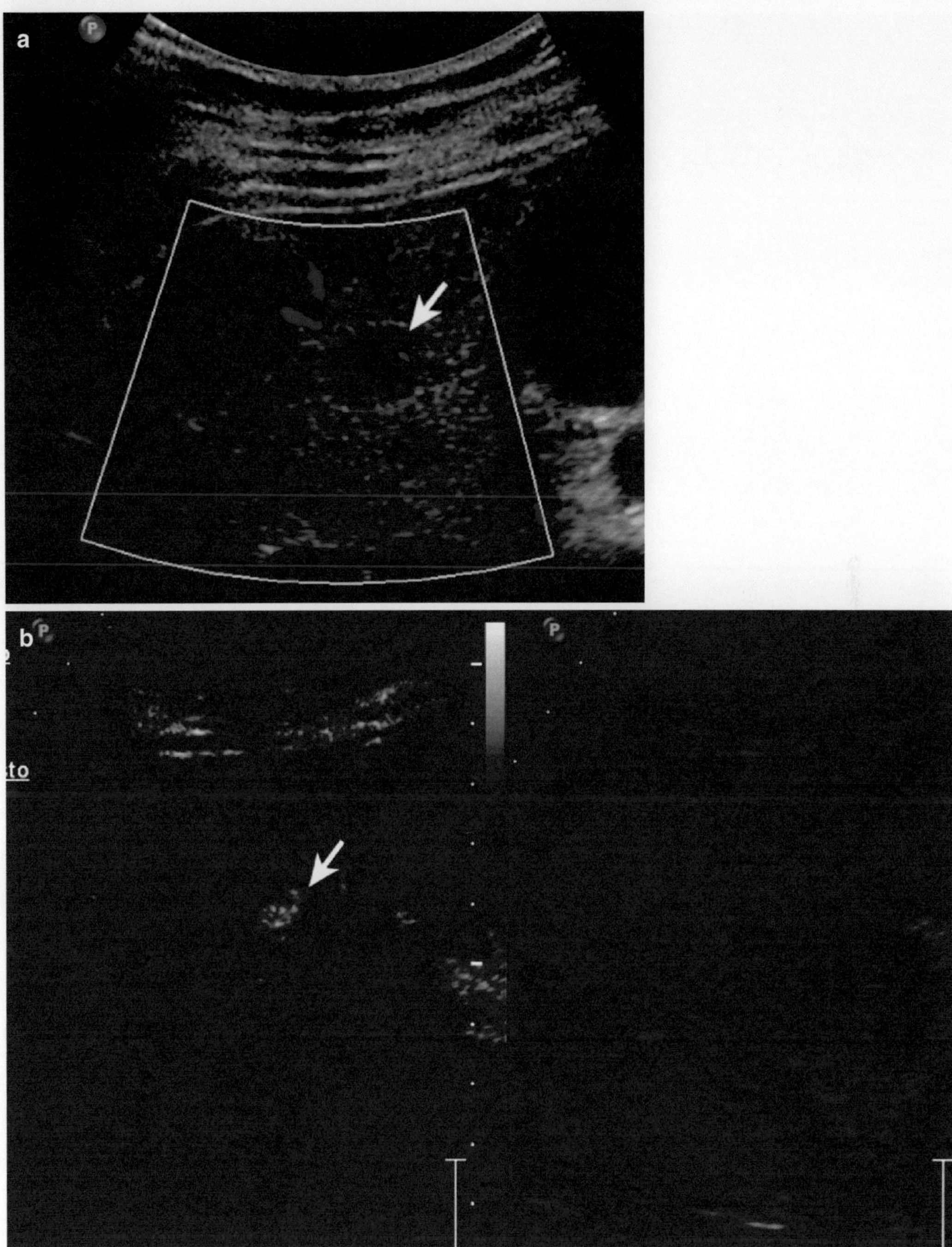

Fig. 2.8 Inside-out hemangioma in a 40-year-old woman. (**a**) Oblique ascending right subcostal baseline image shows a homogeneous hypoechoic 2.2 cm-sized mass in fatty liver with tiny vascular signal at color-Doppler evaluation (*arrow*) in the V hepatic segment; (**b**) in the early arterial phase (20 s after SonoVue injection®), the lesion shows a central enhancing focus (*arrow*); (**c**, **d**) in the portal-venous and late phases, a progressive and complete centrifugal fill-in is shown (*arrows*)

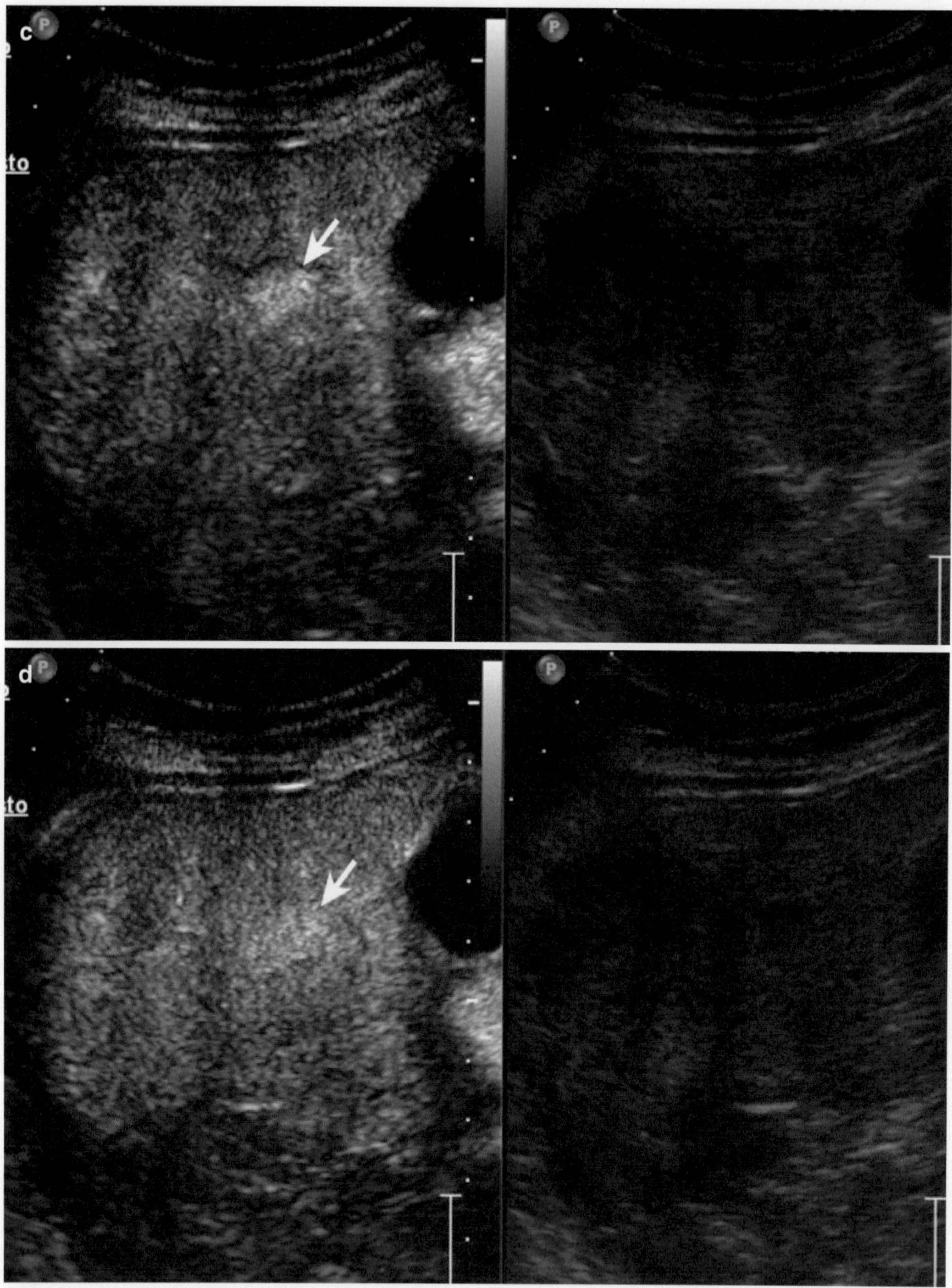

Fig. 2.8 (continued)

2.4 Focal Nodular Hyperplasia

Focal nodular hyperplasia (FNH) is the second-most frequent benign tumor in the liver with an incidence ranging from 1 to 3 %, in most cases incidentally discovered in young women. FNH represents a proliferative response of hepatocytes secondary to a vascular malformation [17]. In fact, the lesion is composed of normal hepatocytes and Kupffer cells separated by fibrous septa with bile ducts and inflammatory cells inside the septa in the absence of classic lobular architecture [18].

Differentiation of FNH from other FLLs is of clinical relevance since surgery is not recommended for asymptomatic patients [19].

Baseline US is not specific for FNH diagnosis because of the absence of specific features. FNH may show different echogenicity, mainly isoechoic (and so difficult to differentiate from the surrounding liver parenchyma), with homogeneous or heterogeneous echotexture and, sometimes, a hyperechoic central area due to a fibrous scar. Color-Doppler and pulsed-Doppler evaluation can demonstrate some peculiar and strongly suggestive feature such as the "spoke-wheel" sign (stellate arterial pattern of vessels within the lesion) or the arterial "feeding vessel" that penetrates inside the lesion from the periphery [20]. Unfortunately, especially in small (<3 cm) or deeply located FNHs, these features are not always evident, and CEUS can provide imaging findings for a correct diagnosis [21]. During the arterial phase, FNH is highly and homogeneously hypervascular, and in the "early arterial phase" just few seconds after the beginning of contrast medium injection, characteristic "spoke-wheel" sign or a "feeding vessel" can be detected [22]. During the portal-venous and late phases, FNH retains contrast medium appearing hyper isoechoic with respect to the surrounding liver parenchyma [23].

In one study, the detection at CEUS of a central star-like fill-in during the early arterial phase was reported to have 100 % specificity for characterizing FNH [24]. But the ability to depict a centrifugal star-like fill-in is strictly dependent on the timing of scanning, and CEUS, representing a real-time imaging study, is well suited to this purpose, more than interval delay techniques as CT and MRI [25].

Moreover, a constantly hypoechoic central area representing a fibrous scar may be depicted at CEUS. So color-/power-Doppler analysis and CEUS findings are essential for the final diagnosis [26, 27].

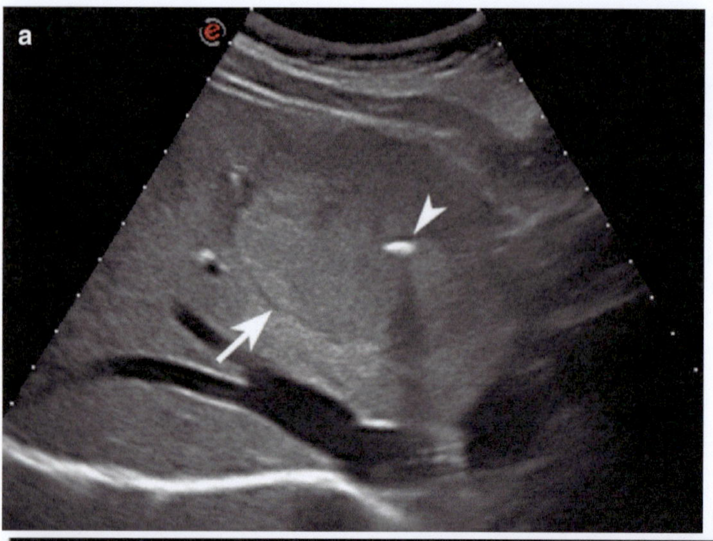

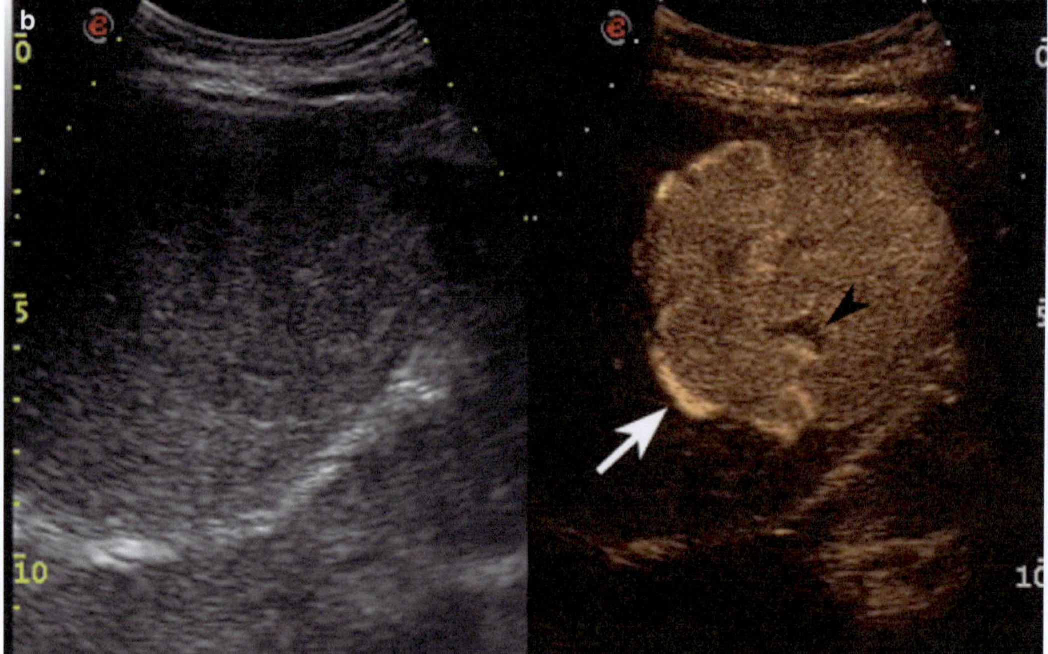

Fig. 2.9 Focal nodular hyperplasia in a 31-year-old woman. (**a**) Baseline US image shows an isoechoic lesion sized 7.2 cm in the VIII hepatic segment (*arrow*) with small calcification in the central portion (*arrowhead*). (**b**) At CEUS, the lesion appears highly and homogeneously hypervascular in the arterial phase (*arrow*) showing a sustained contrast enhancement during the remaining portal-venous (**c**) and late (**d**) phases, except for a central constantly avascular area corresponding to the "central scar"(*arrowheads*)

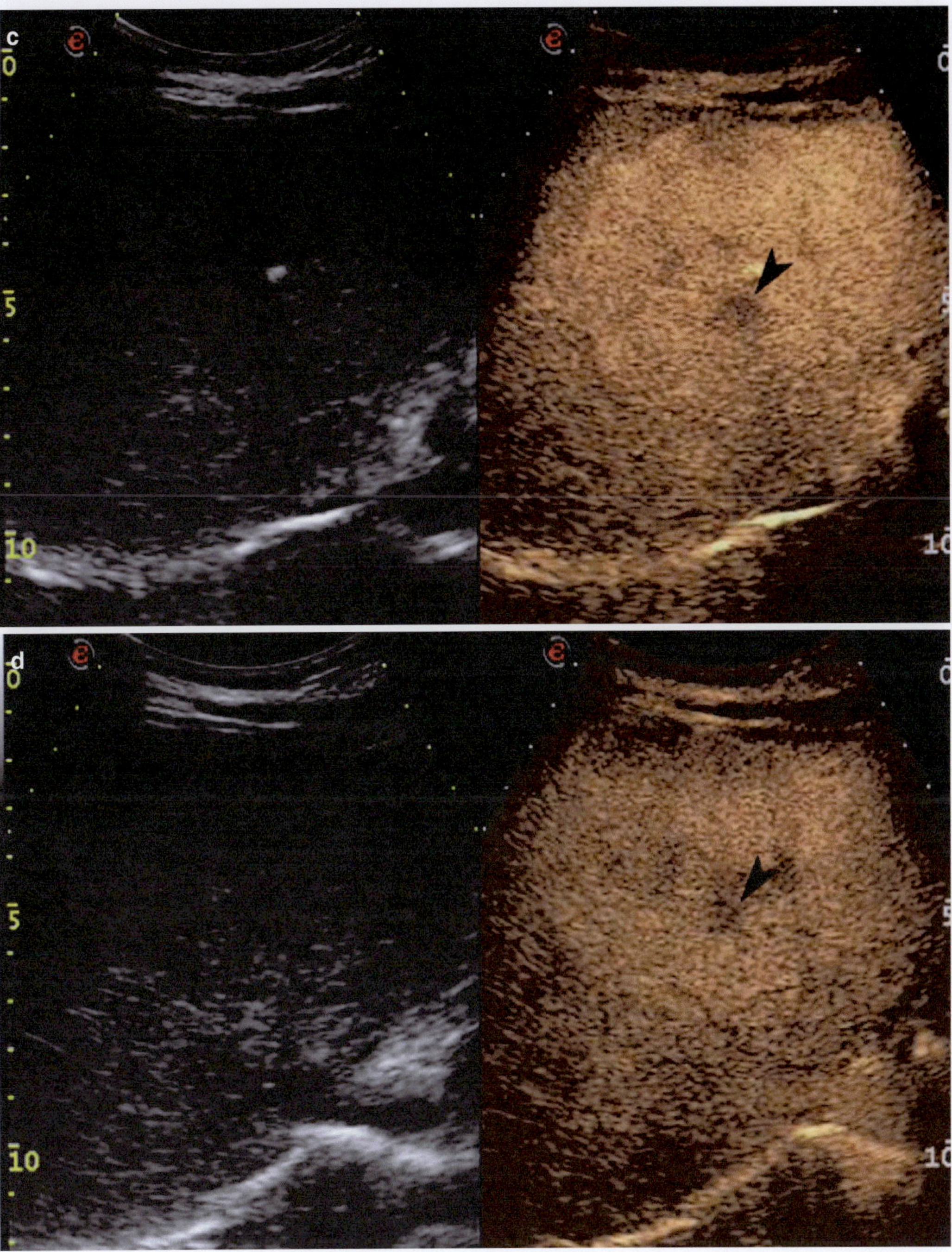

Fig. 2.9 (continued)

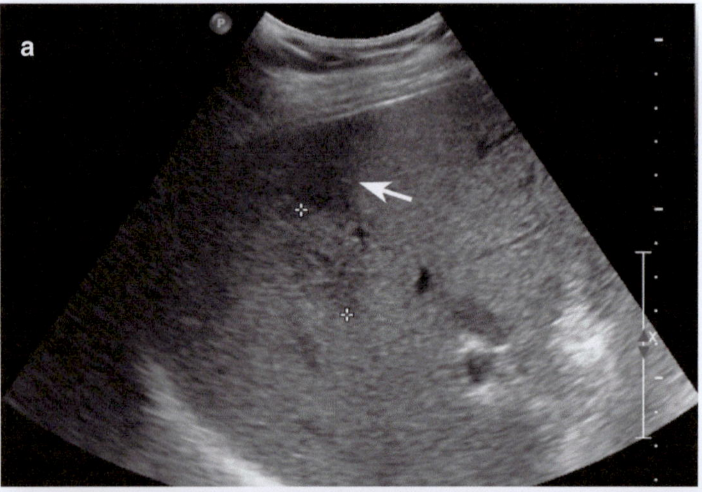

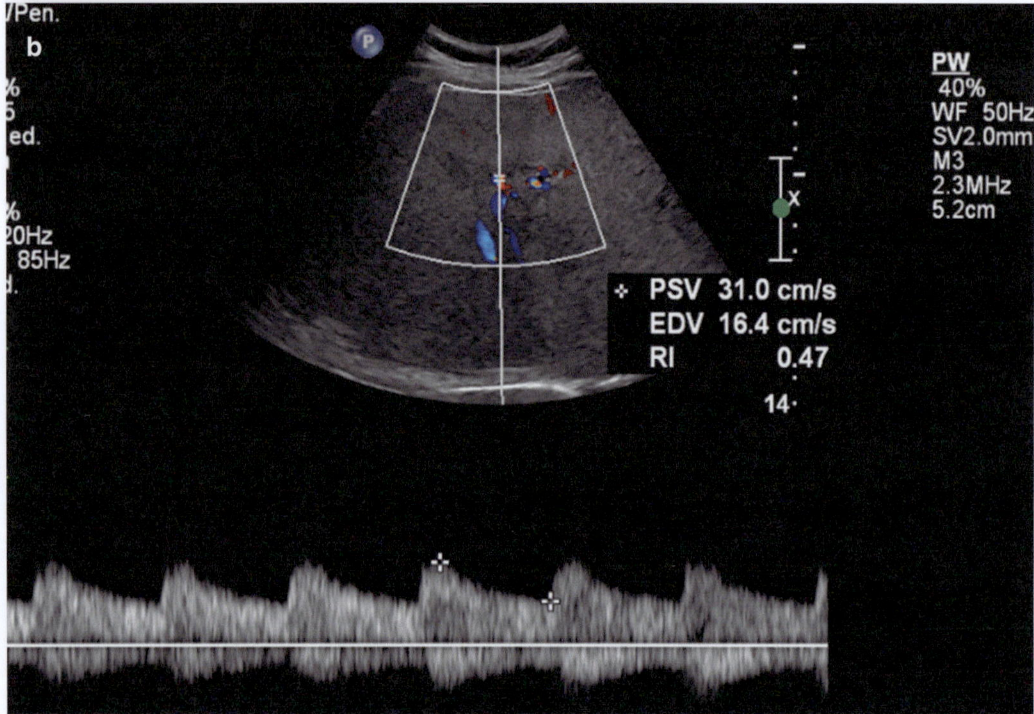

Fig. 2.10 Focal nodular hyperplasia and focal fatty sparing. (**a**) Baseline US shows a 3.4-cm slightly hypoechoic lesion located in segment V (*calipers*) with intralesional arterial signal at pulsed-Doppler evaluation (**b**). Adjacent to the above mentioned lesion, a hypoechoic area with ill-defined margins is also appreciable in **a** (*arrow*). (**c**) At CEUS in the arterial phase, the lesion shows a clear-cut and homogeneous contrast enhancement (*arrow*) except for a small central hypoechoic area representing the central scar (*black arrowhead*). A feeding vessel is evident too (*white arrowhead*). The lesion presents sustained enhancement in the portal-venous (**d**) and late (**e**) phases (*arrows*). The area surrounding the FNH is not evident throughout the vascular study suggesting a pseudolesion (focal fatty sparing)

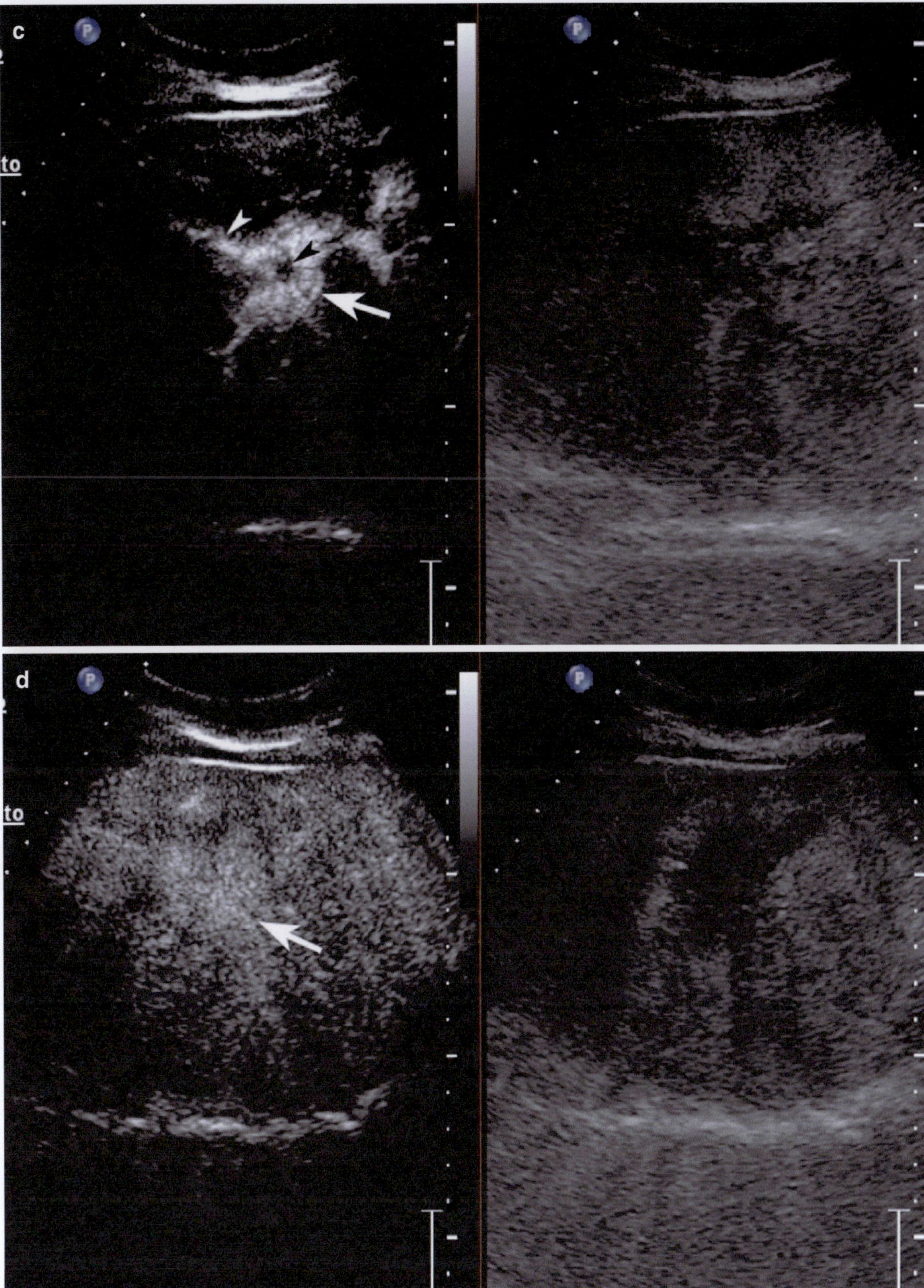

Fig. 2.10 (continued)

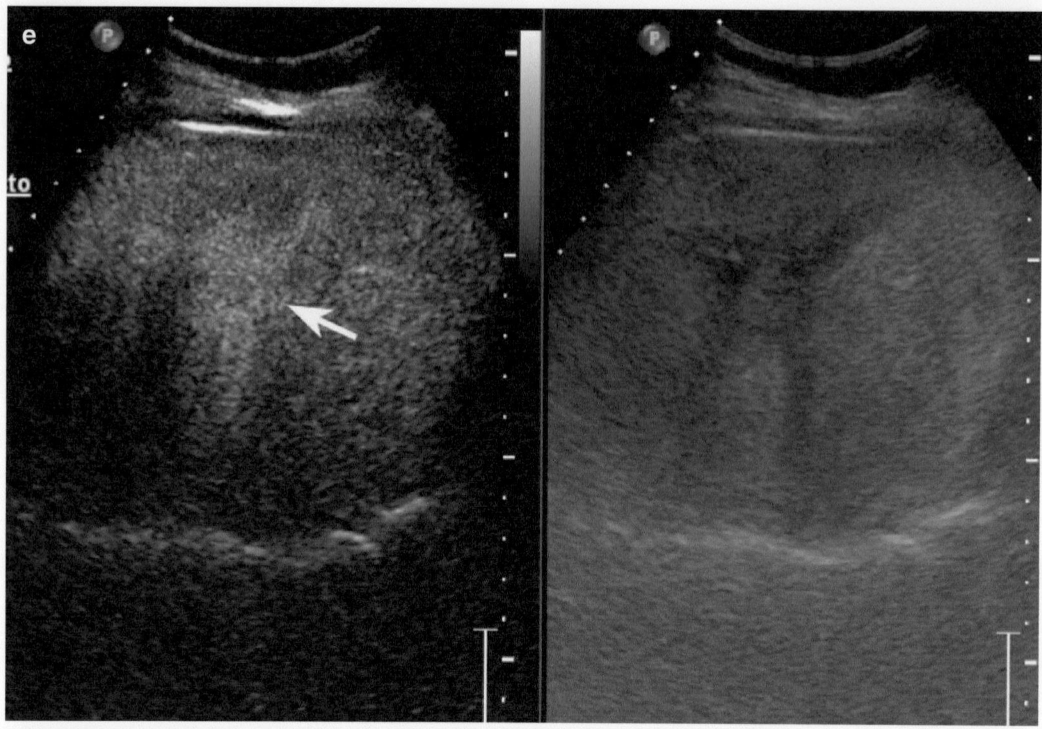

Fig. 2.10 (continued)

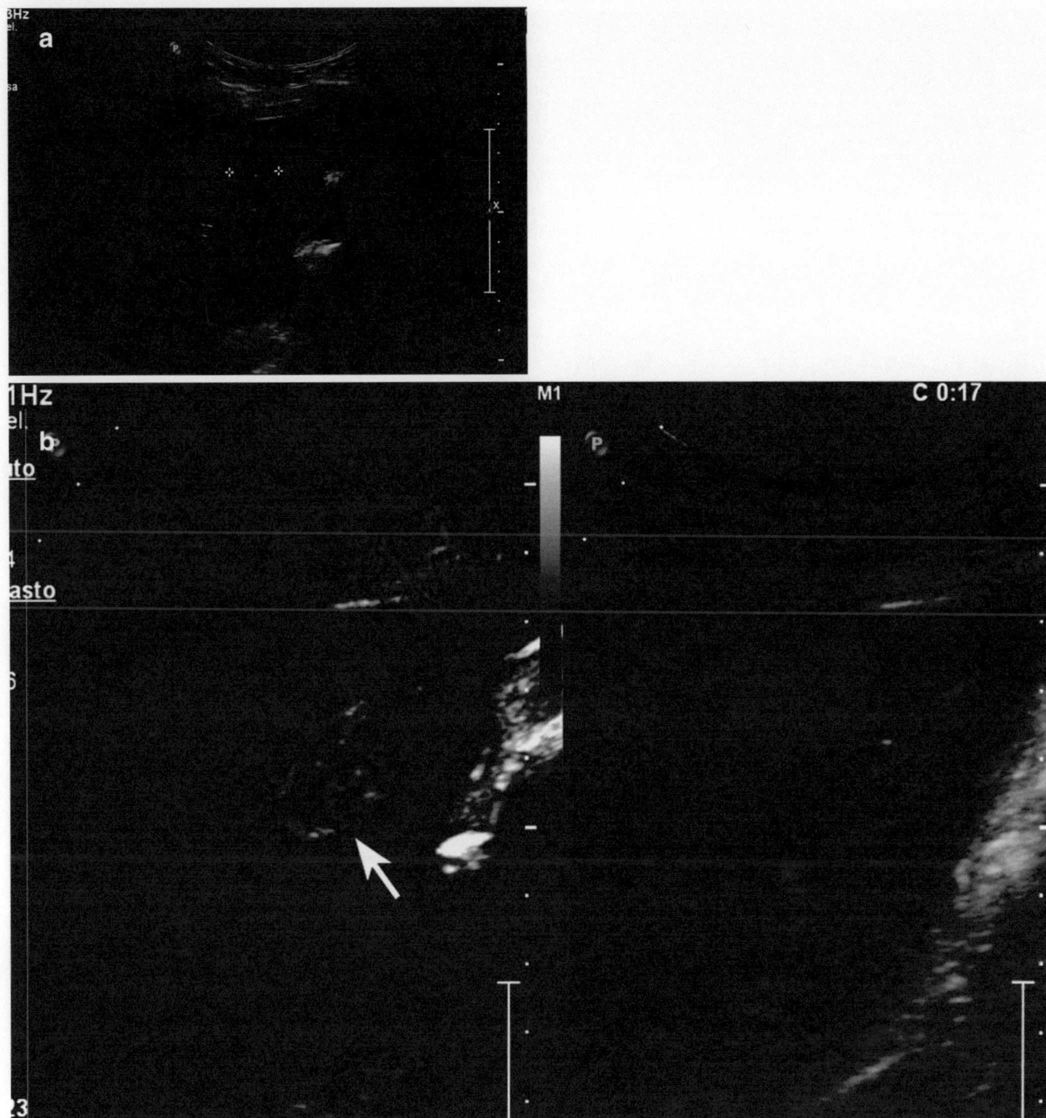

Fig. 2.11 Focal nodular hyperplasia in a 28-year-old woman. (**a**) Baseline US shows a 1.7-cm slightly hyperechoic lesion located in segment V (*calipers*). (**b**) CEUS depicts the spoke-wheel sign in the early arterial phase (*arrow*). (**c**) In the late arterial phase, the lesion shows a clear-cut and homogeneous contrast enhancement (*arrow*) (**d**) The lesion is isovascular with respect to the surrounding liver parenchyma in the late phase

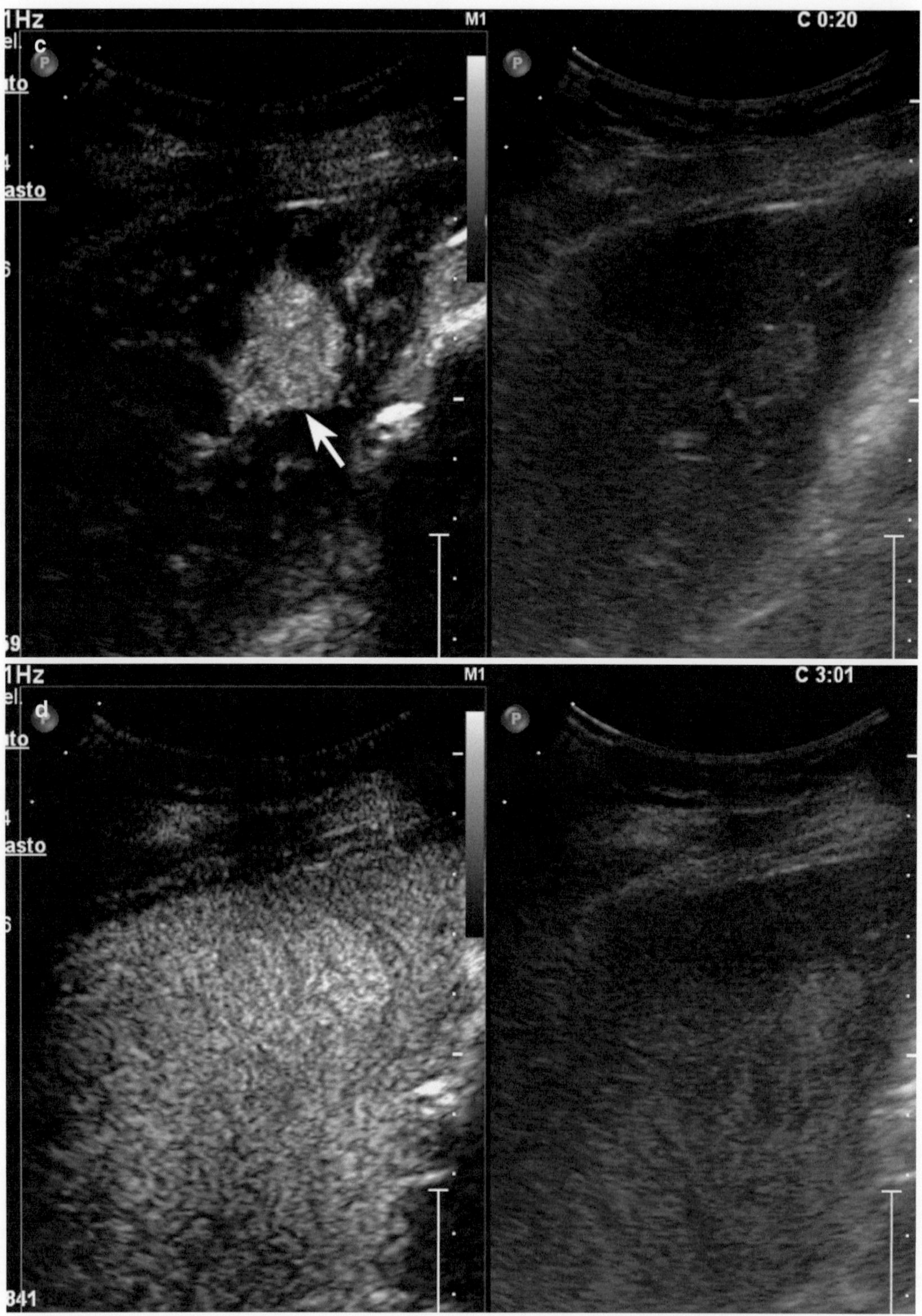

Fig. 2.11 (continued)

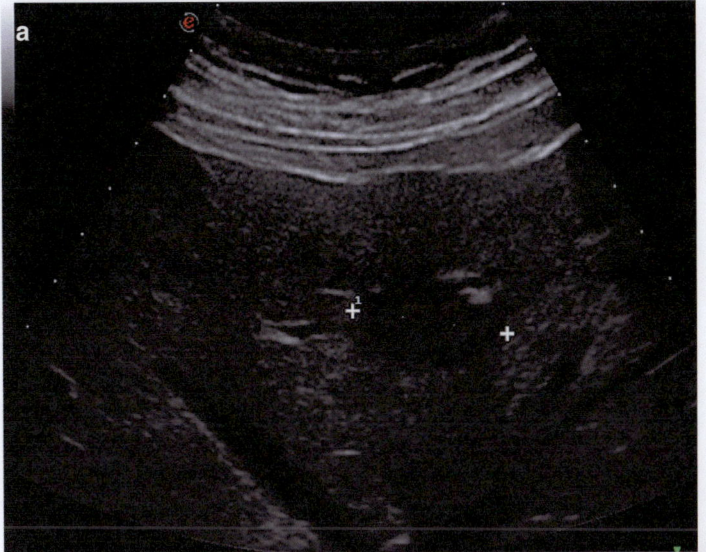

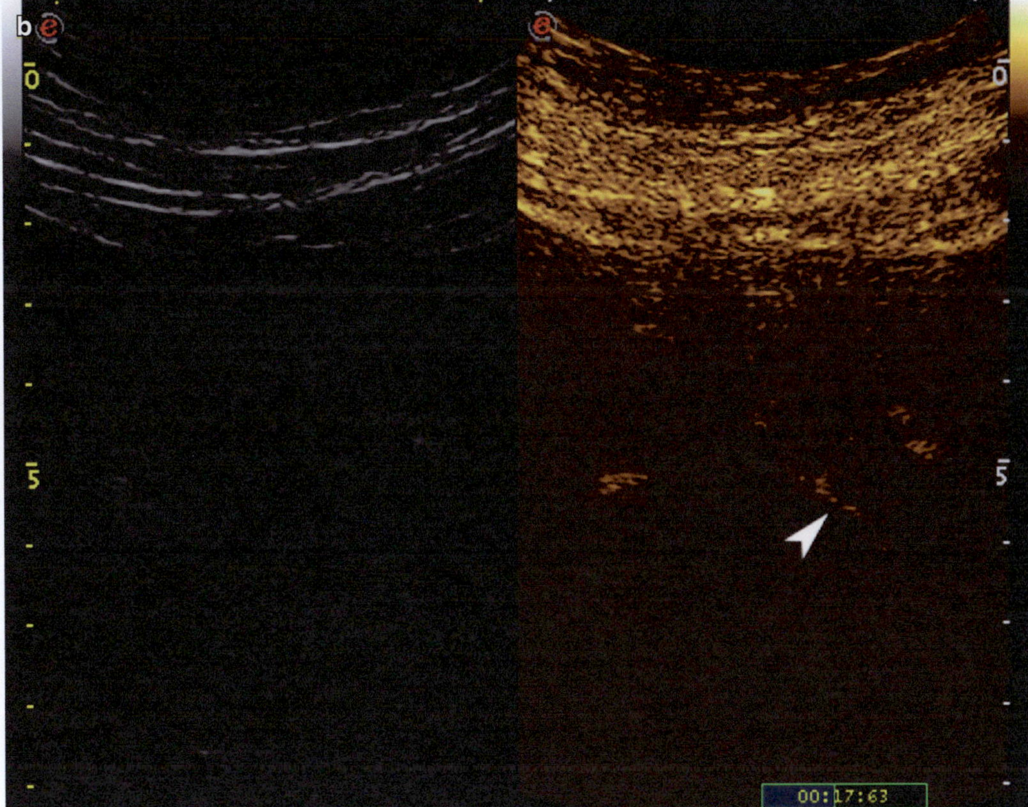

Fig. 2.12 Focal nodular hyperplasia in a 35-year-old man. (**a**) Baseline US shows a 3 cm-sized hypoechoic lesion located in segment IV in fatty liver (*calipers*). (**b**) At CEUS, in the early arterial phase, a feeding vessel is appreciable (*arrowhead*). (**c**) During the late arterial phase, the lesion shows a clear-cut and homogeneous contrast enhancement (*arrow*) and presents isoechoic aspect during the extended portal-venous phase (**d**)

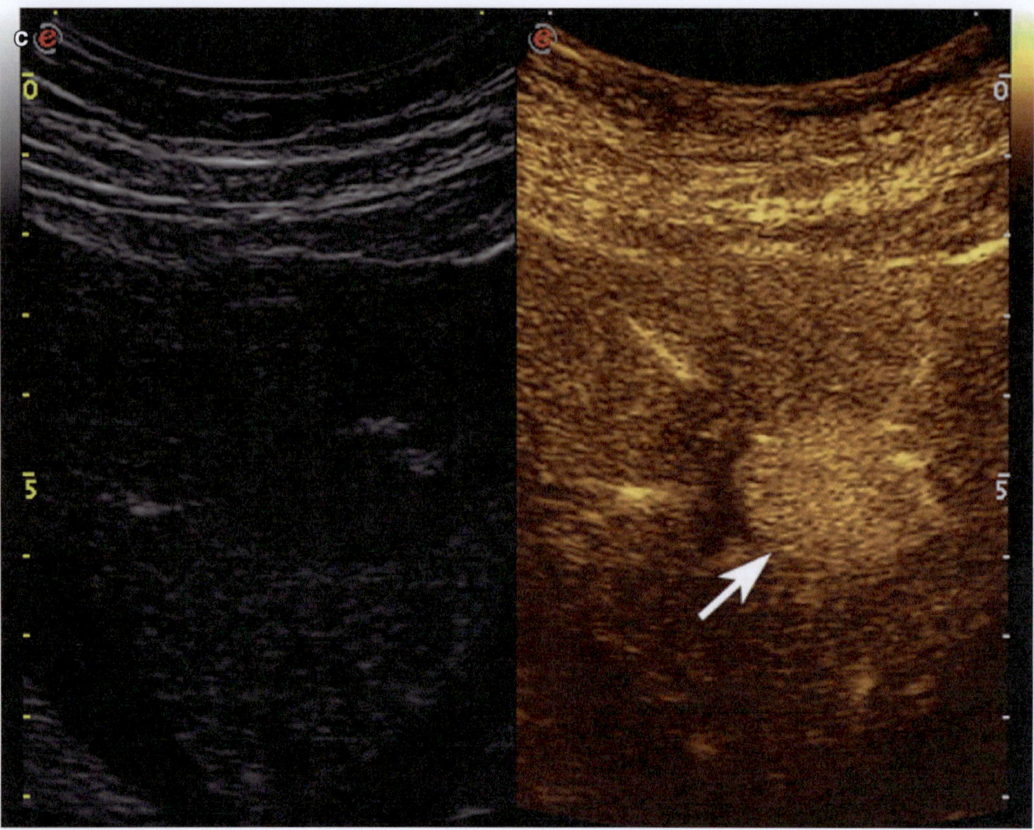

Fig. 2.12 (continued)

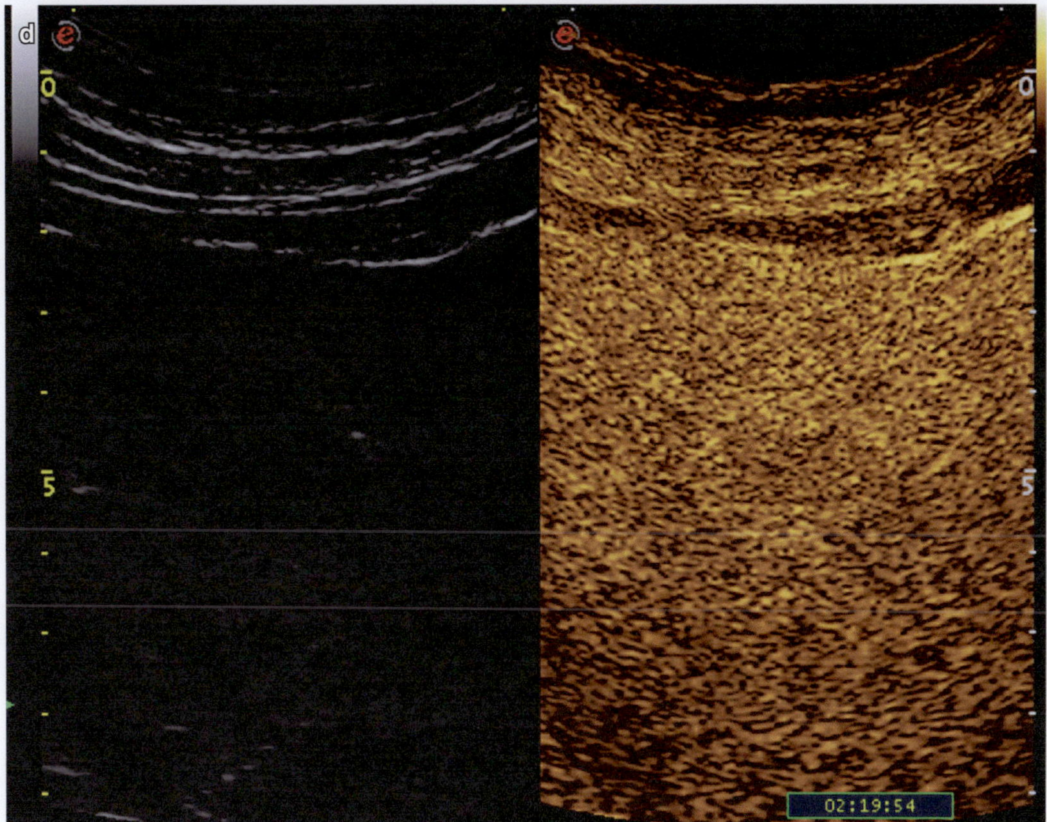

Fig. 2.12   (continued)

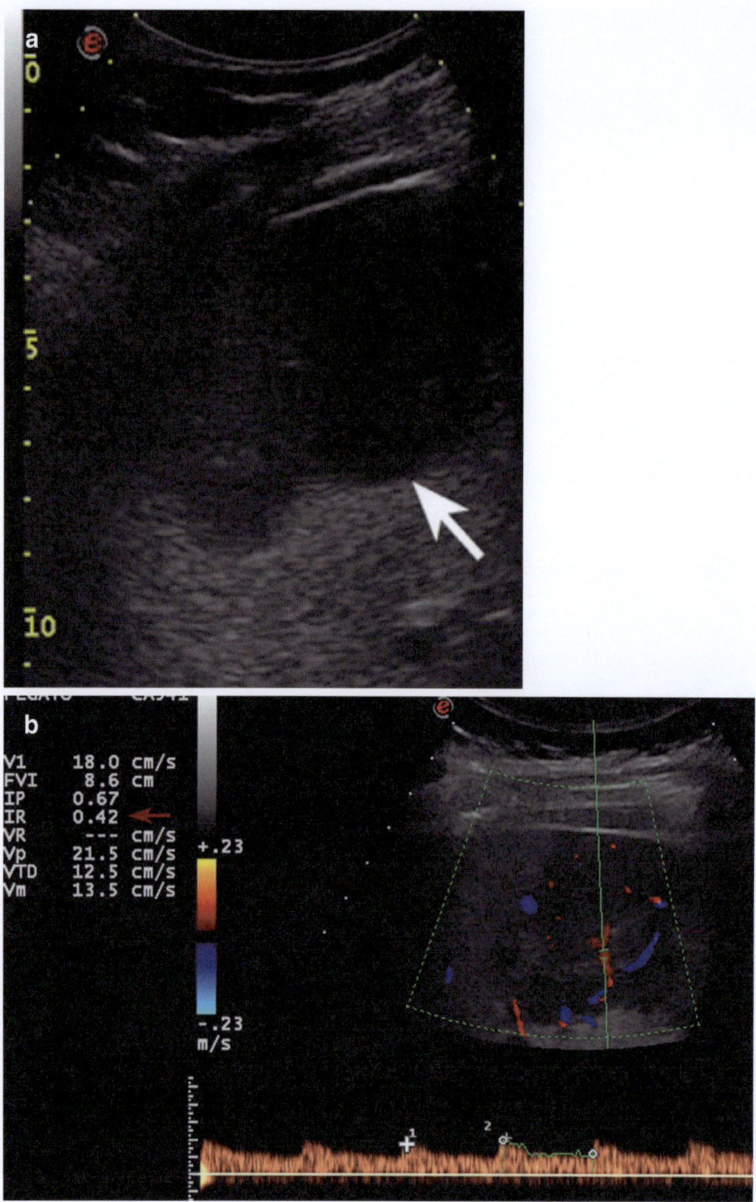

Fig. 2.13 Focal nodular hyperplasia in a 35-year-old woman. (**a**) Baseline US image shows a 7.8-cm-sized highly hypoechoic lesion located in segment VIII (*arrow*). (**b**) At color/pulsed-Doppler evaluation, the spoke-wheel sign is evident with low resistance index arterial signal (*red arrow*). (**c**) CEUS confirms the spoke-wheel aspect (*arrow*) in the early arterial phase. (**d**) In the late arterial phase, the lesion shows a clear-cut and homogeneous contrast enhancement (*arrow*) and appears to be isovascular with respect to the surrounding liver parenchyma in the portal venous (**e**) and late phases (*arrows*) (**f**)

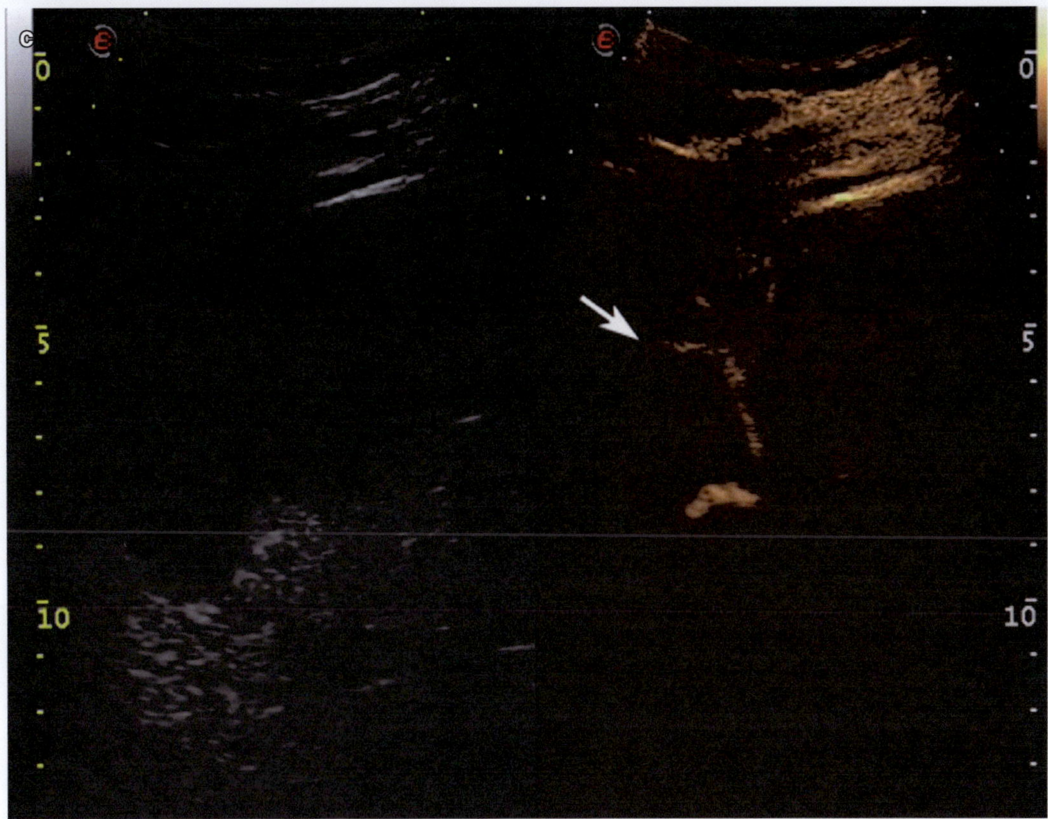

Fig. 2.13 (continued)

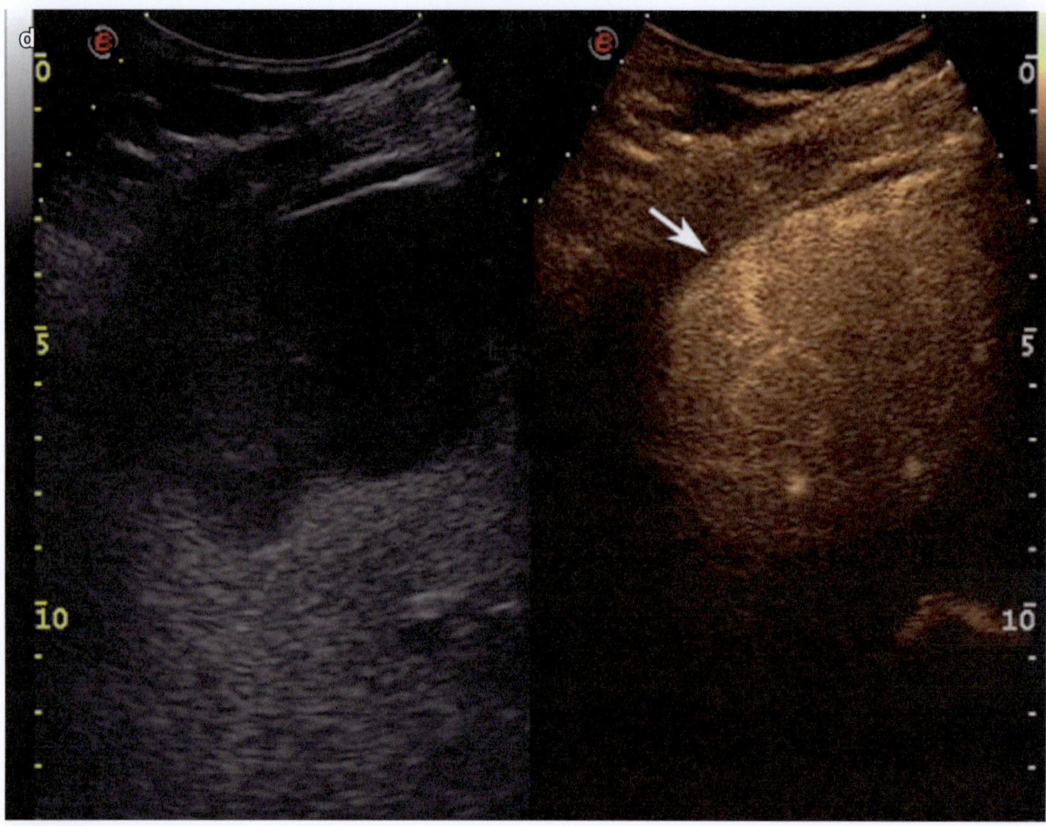

Fig. 2.13 (continued)

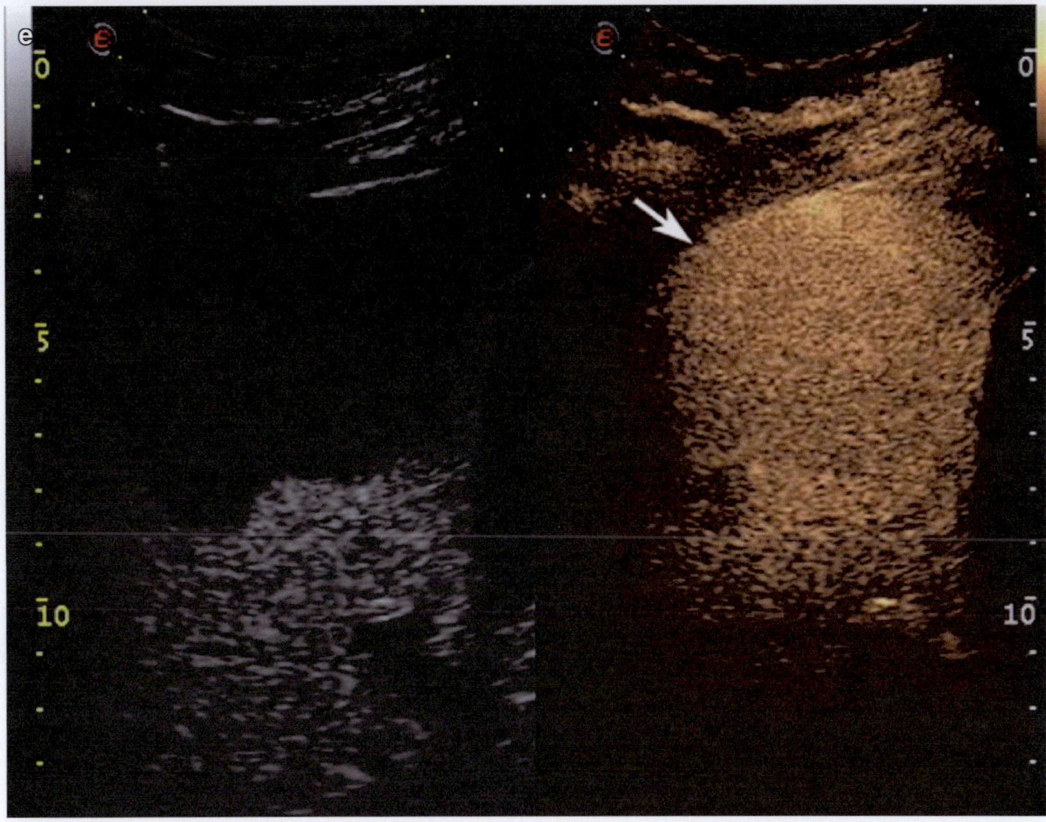

Fig. 2.13 (continued)

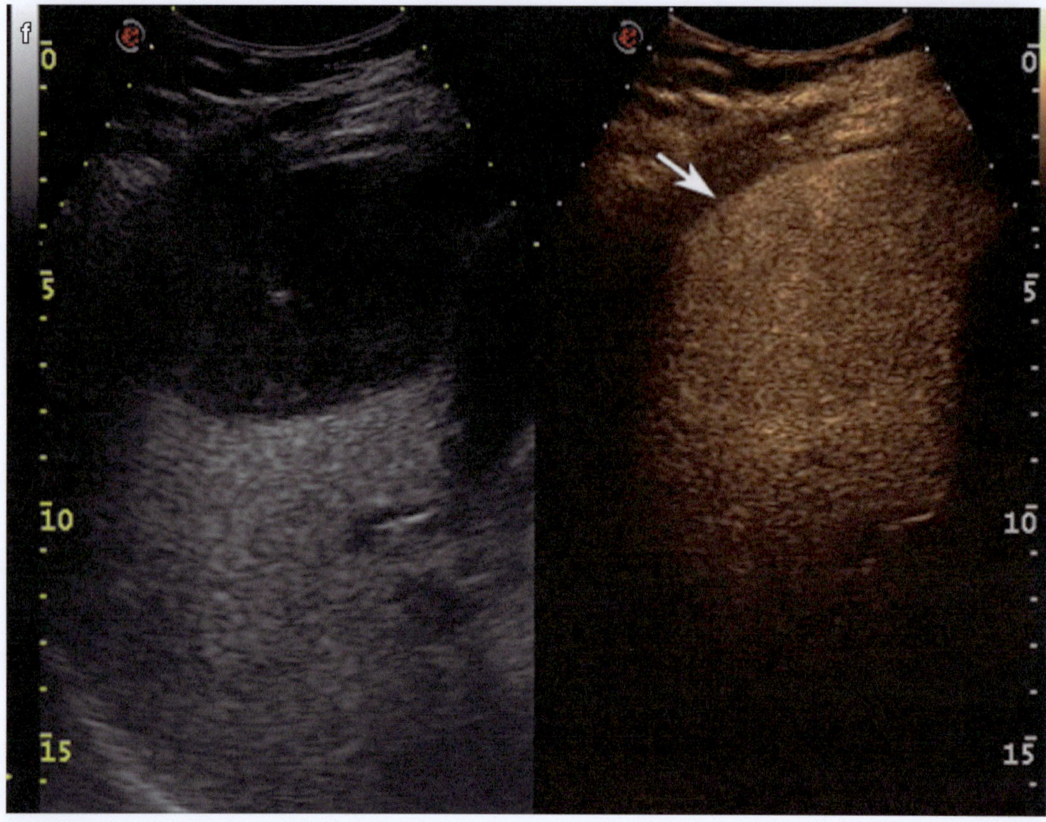

Fig. 2.13 (continued)

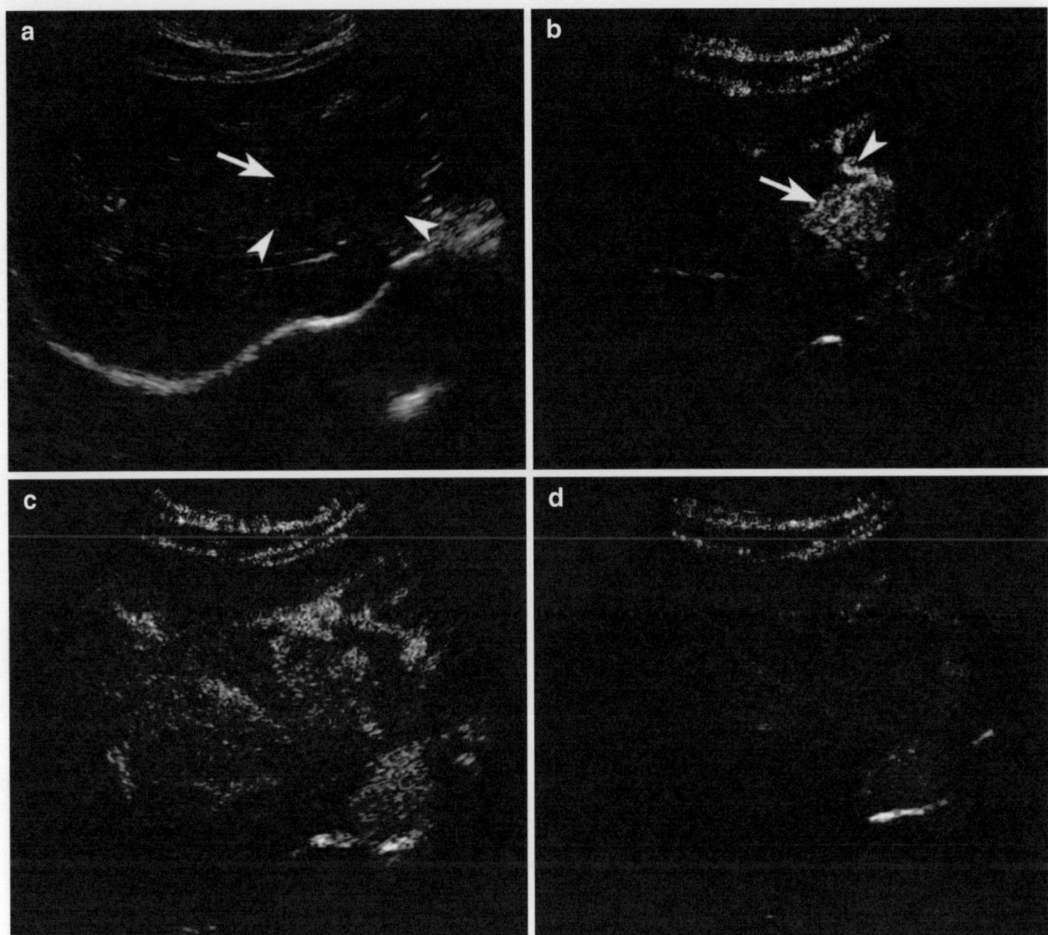

Fig. 2.14 Focal nodular hyperplasia in a 41-year-old woman. (**a**) Baseline US shows a 2.4 cm-sized isoechoic lesion located in the IV segment (*arrow*) between middle and left suprahepatic veins (*arrowheads*). (**b**) At CEUS, during the arterial phase, the lesion presents a strong and homogeneous enhancement (*arrow*), and a feeding vessel is appreciable in the upper side (*arrowhead*). (**c**, **d**) The lesion becomes isovascular with respect to the surrounding liver parenchyma during the portal-venous (**c**) and late (**d**) phases

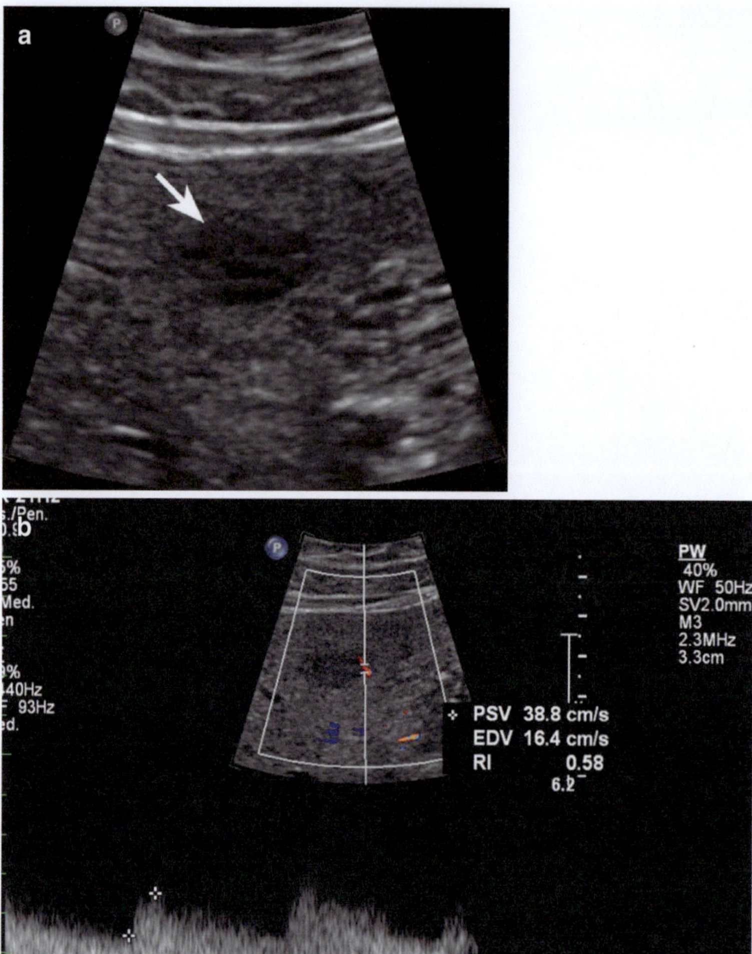

Fig. 2.15 FNH in a 46-year-old man. (**a**) Baseline US shows a 1.5 cm-sized moderately hypoechoic lesion located in the V segment (*arrow*). (**b**) A peripheral arterial vessel is evident at color- and pulsed-Doppler. (**c**) At CEUS, during the arterial phase, the lesion presents a strong and homogeneous enhancement (*arrow*). (**d**, **e**) The lesion maintains slightly hypervascular aspect during the portal-venous phase (*arrows*) (**d**) and appears isoechoic during the late phase (**e**). (**f**) Islice 3D reconstruction during the arterial phase confirms a strong and homogeneous lesion enhancement and confirms a feeding vessel in the lateral portion (*arrowheads*)

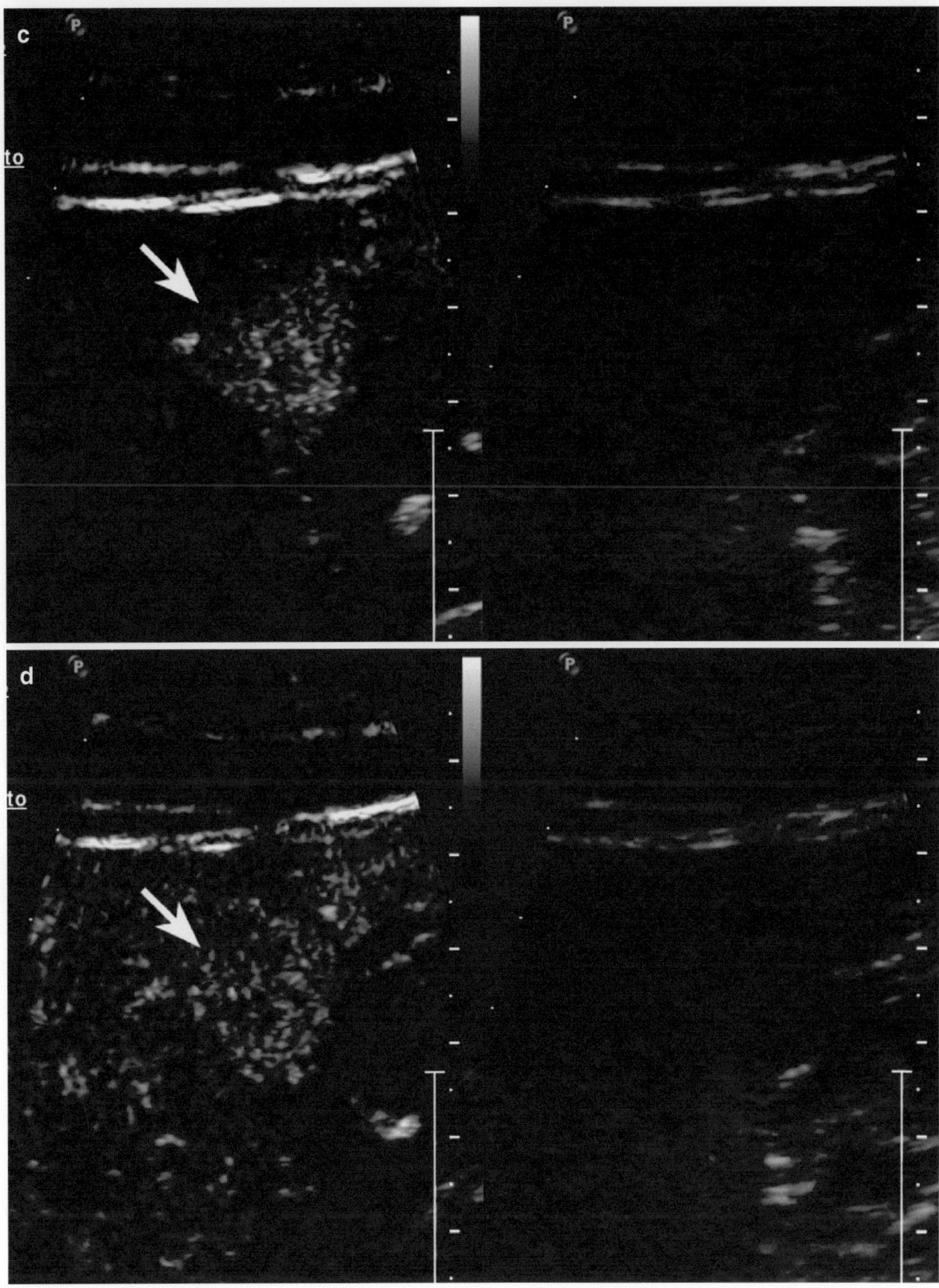

Fig. 2.15 (continued)

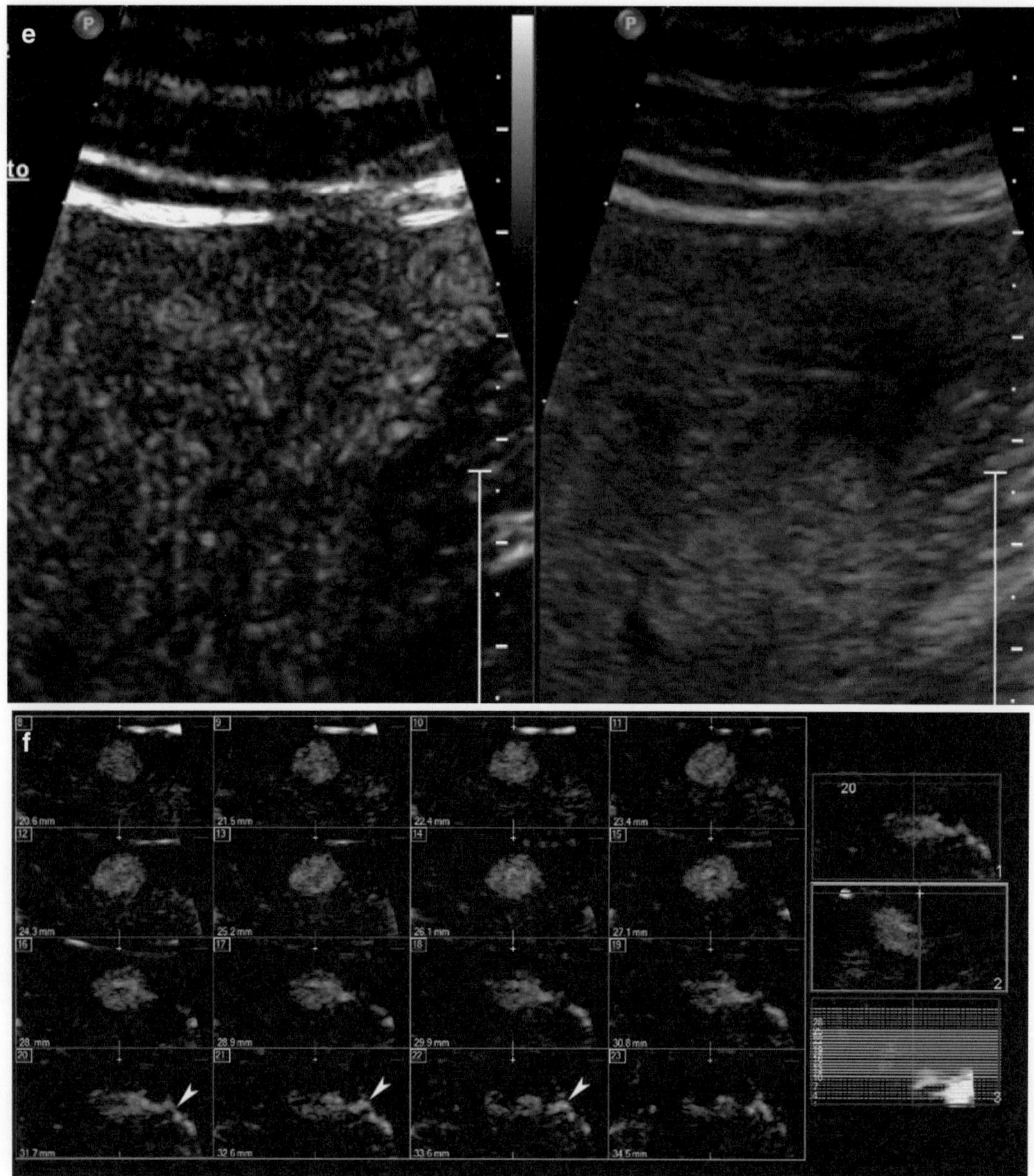

Fig. 2.15 (continued)

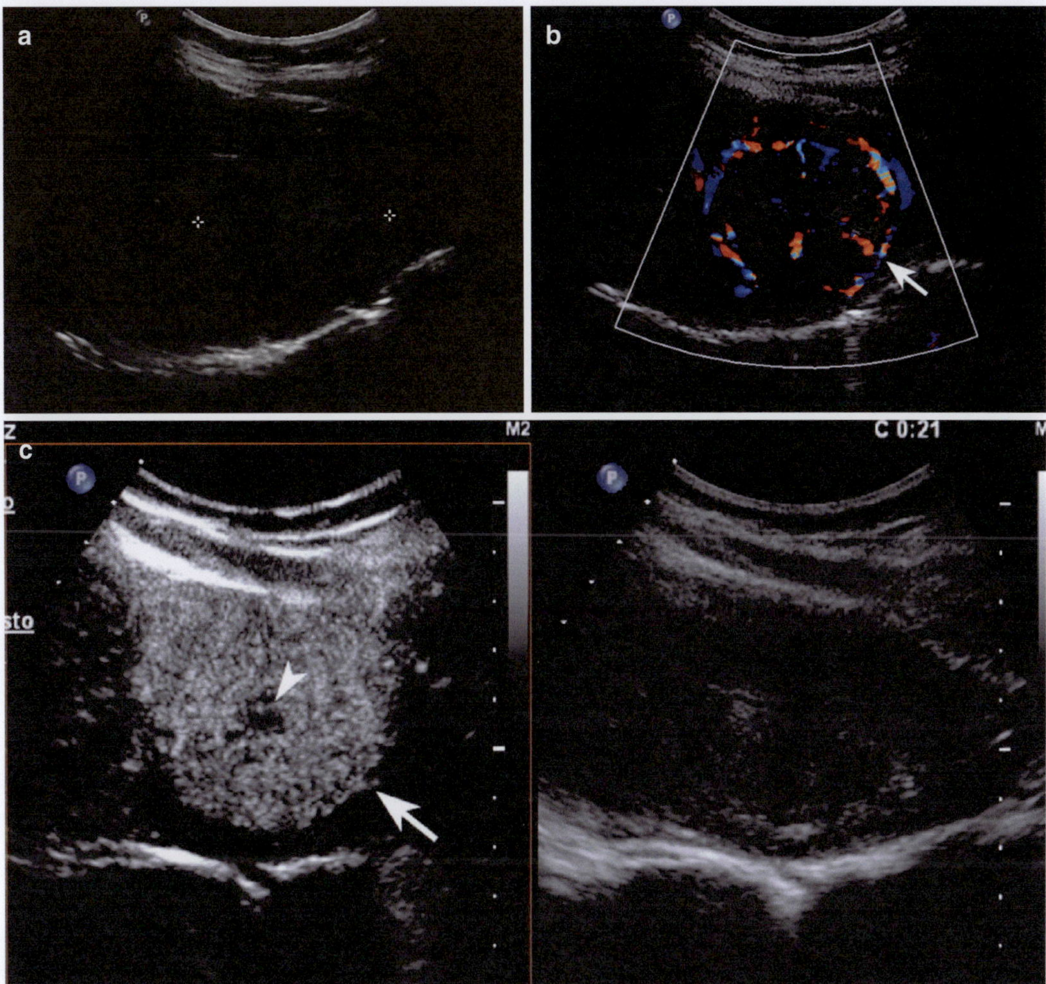

Fig. 2.16 Focal nodular hyperplasia in a 49-year-old woman. (**a**) Baseline US image shows a slightly inhomogeneous hyperechoic lesion sized 5.4 cm in the VIII hepatic segment (*calipers*). (**b**) At color-Doppler evaluation, spoke-wheel sign is evident (*arrow*). (**c**) At CEUS, the lesion appears highly and homogeneously hypervascular in the arterial phase (*arrow*) showing a sustained contrast enhancement during the remaining portal-venous (**d**) and late (**e**) phases (*arrows*), except for a central constantly avascular area corresponding to the "central scar"(*arrowheads*)

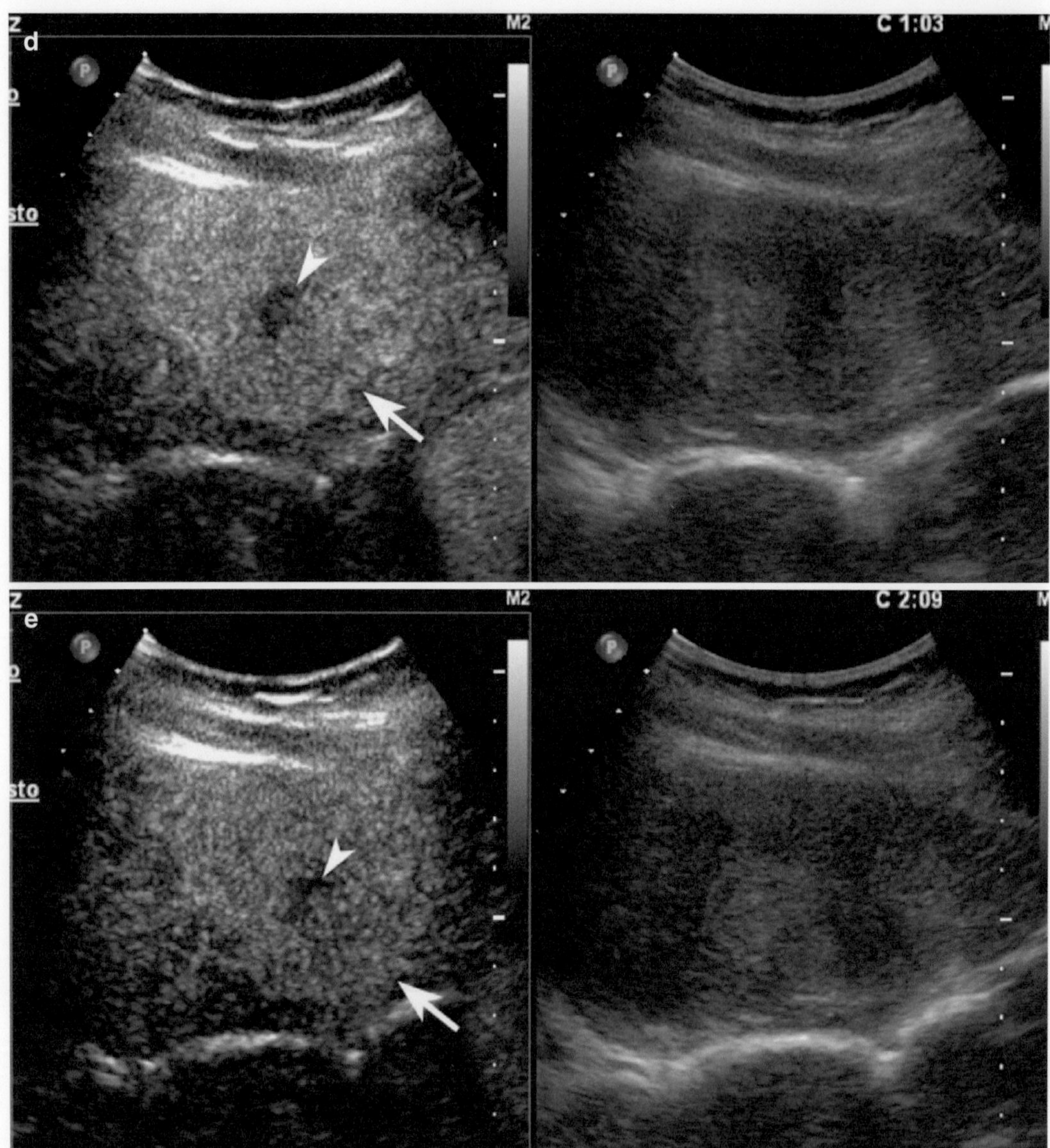

Fig. 2.16 (continued)

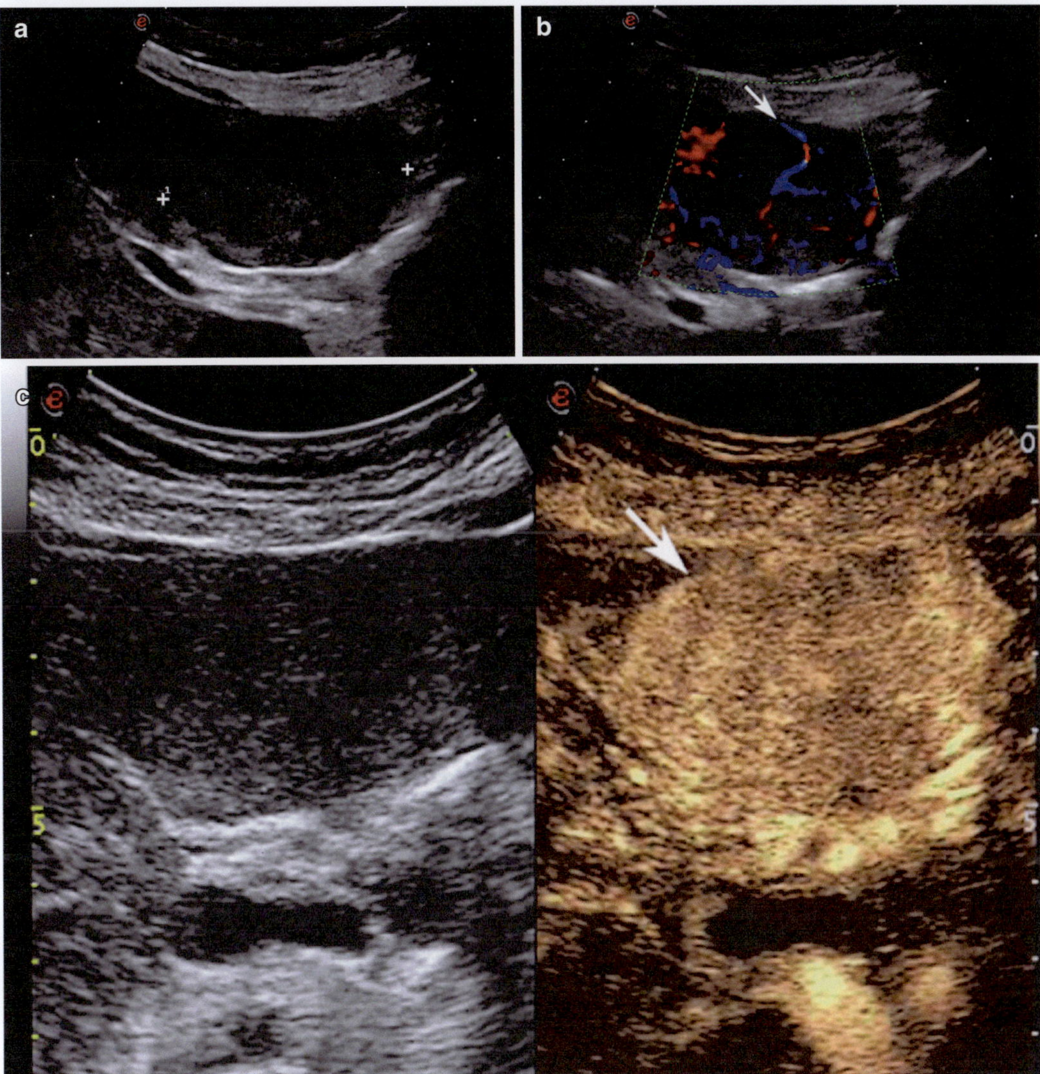

Fig. 2.17 Focal nodular hyperplasia in a 32-year-old woman. (**a**) Baseline US shows a 5.6 cm-sized isoechoic lesion located in segment IV (*calipers*). (**b**) Color-Doppler evaluation shows the spoke-wheel sign (*arrow*). (**c**) At CEUS, in the arterial phase, the lesion shows a marked and homogeneous contrast enhancement (*arrow*) and presents isoechoic aspect during, respectively, the portal-venous (**d**) and late (**e**) phases (*arrows*)

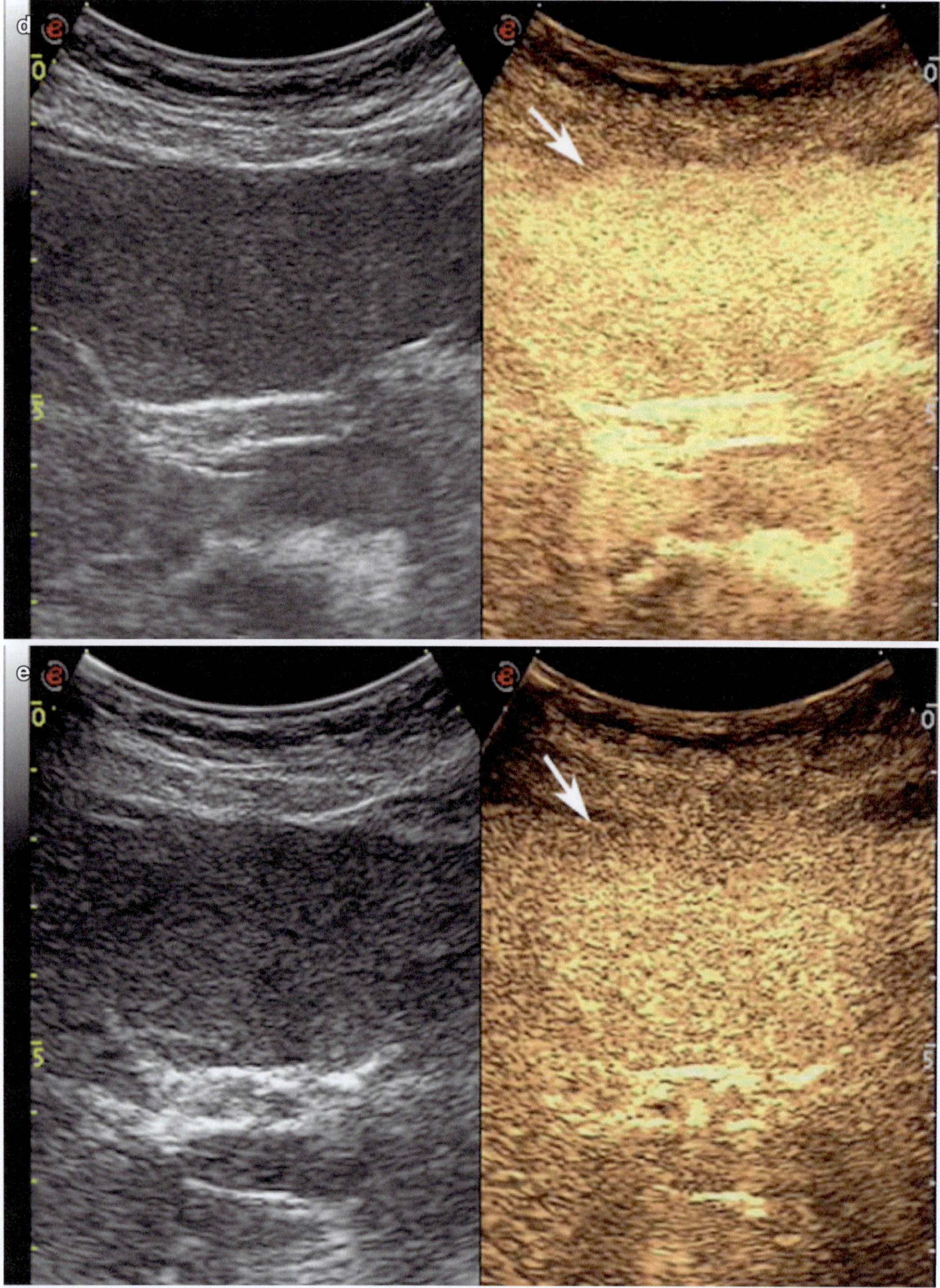

Fig. 2.17 (continued)

2.5 **Hepatocellular Adenoma**

Hepatocellular adenoma (HA) is a rare hepatic lesion, most commonly discovered in young women and closely associated with the assumption of oral contraceptives, anabolic steroid, and glycogen storage disease.

HA consists of normal hepatocytes with a variable rate of fat and glycogen, fibrous tissue and large sinusoids related to a high risk of bleeding especially in large lesions. Moreover, malignant degeneration is possible. Hence, a correct diagnosis is mandatory since surgical resection is advised mainly for HA larger than 4 cm [28–30].

At grayscale US, HA can present various appearances with homogeneous or inhomogeneous echotexure depending on the size or the presence of thrombotic–hemorrhagic phenomena. Colour- and power-Doppler are not specific too.

On the basis of literature papers and our experience, HA (hepatocyte nuclear factor 1α (HNF1α)-inactivated subtype) usually presents as homogeneously or heterogeneously moderately hypervascular with a mixed or centripetal filling during the arterial phase and may appear indistinguishable from the surrounding hepatic parenchyma in the extended portal-venous phase [31].

Nevertheless, in a not-negligible number of cases, HA (inflammatory subtype) may present hypovascular aspect in the extended portal venous phase, whereas larger lesions, with mixed echotexture or even hemorrhagic, may show an inhomogeneous, mainly peripheral, contrast enhancement after SonoVue® injection [32, 33].

In the abovementioned cases, differentiate HA from malignant lesions is quite hard, and further imaging workup or even biopsy may be required [34].

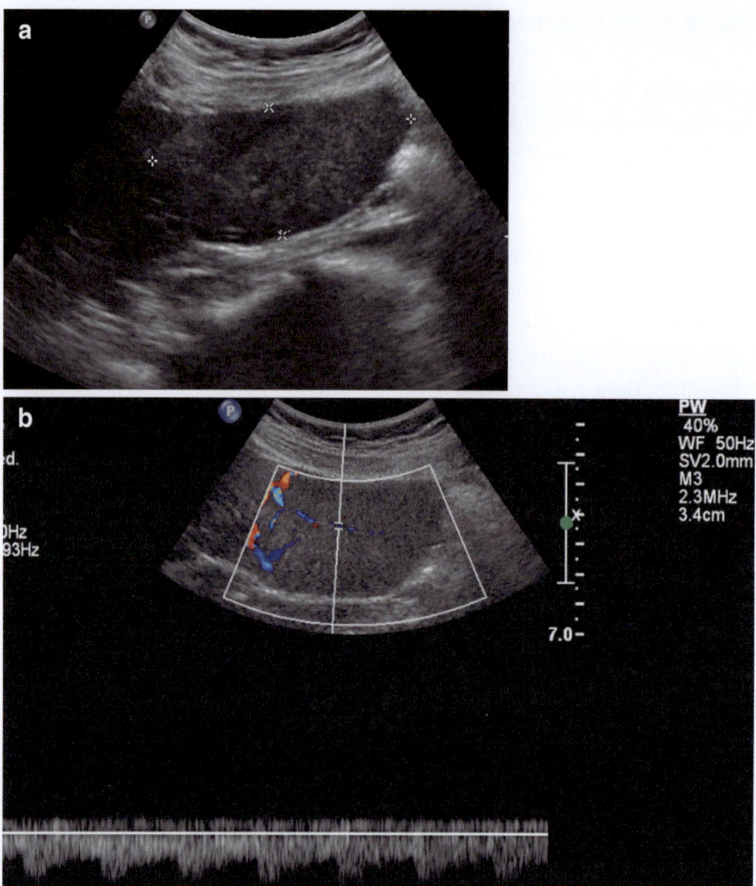

Fig. 2.18 Biopsy-proved hepatocellular adenoma in a 37-year-old woman. (**a**) Baseline US image shows a slightly hyperechoic lesion sized 7.7 cm in the left lobe (*calipers*). (**b**) At pulsed-Doppler evaluation, some arterial vessel is evident within the mass. (**c**) At CEUS, the lesion appears highly and homogeneously hypervascular in the arterial phase showing a sustained contrast enhancement during the remaining portal-venous (**d**) and late (**e**) phases (*arrows*)

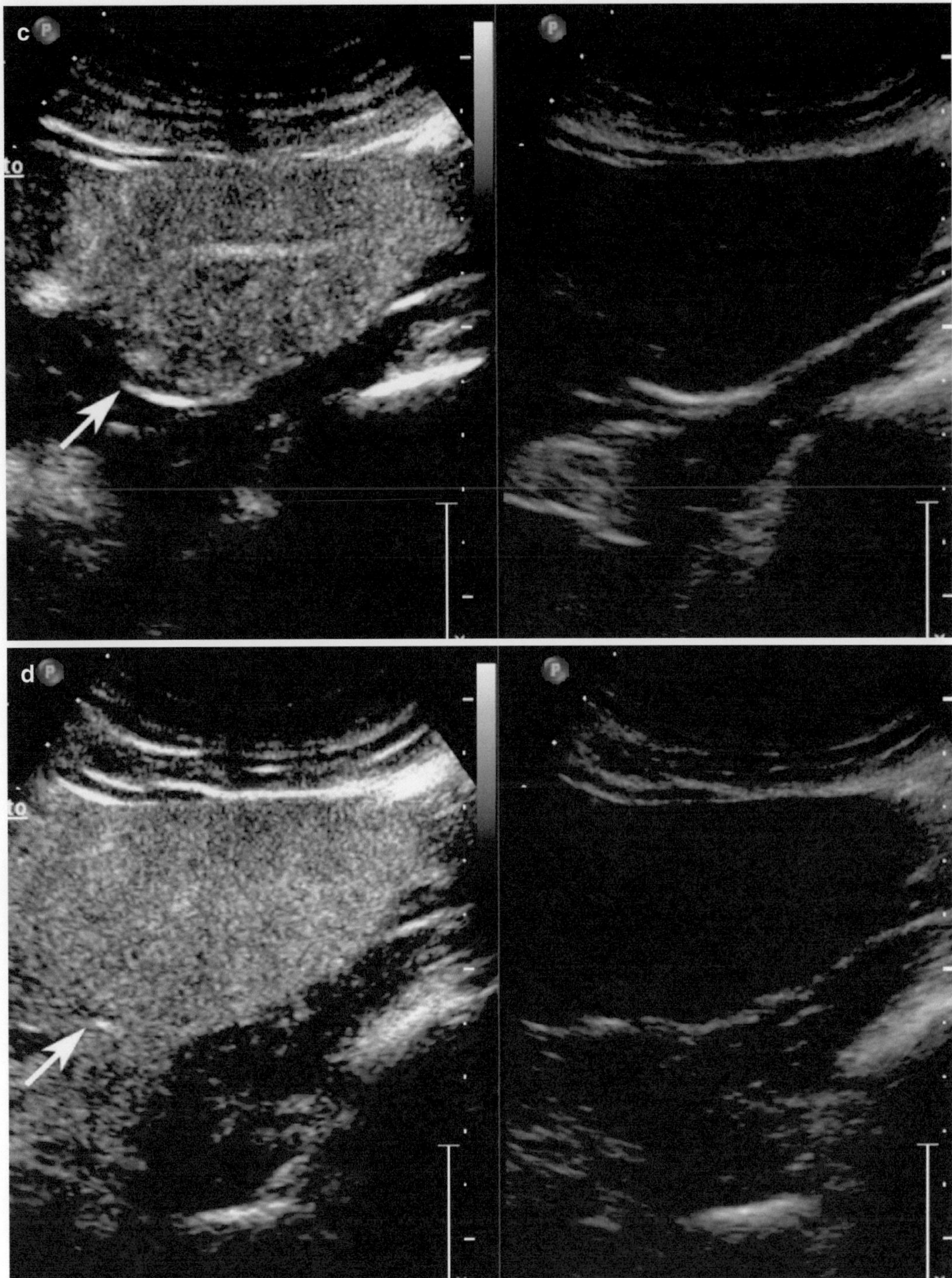

Fig. 2.18 (continued)

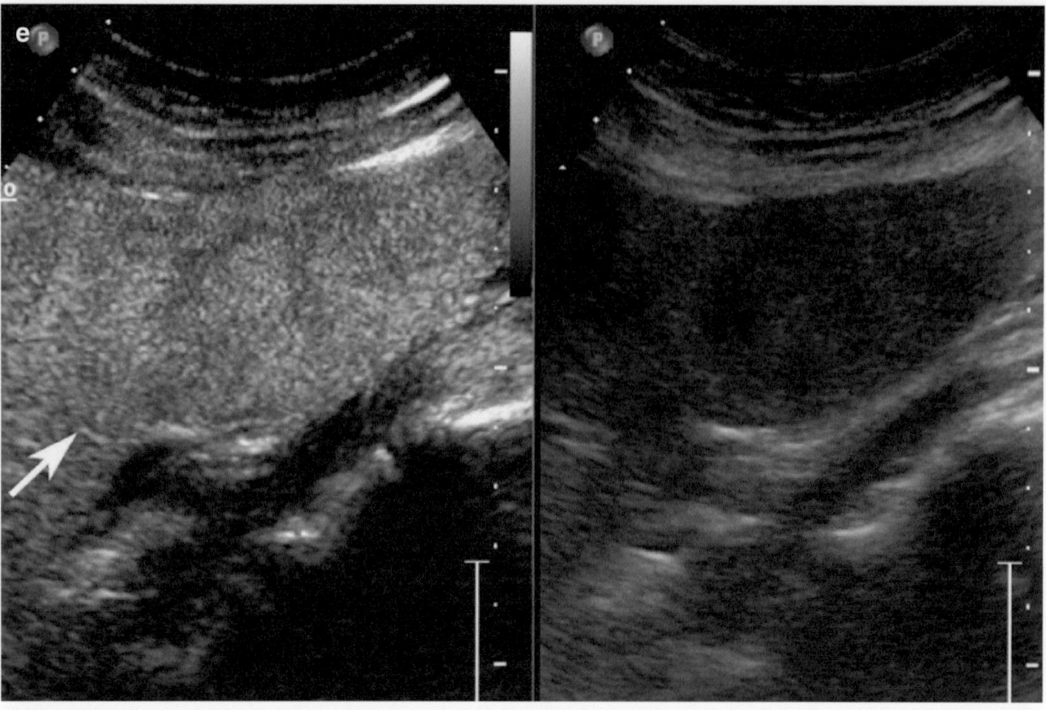

Fig. 2.18 (continued)

2.6 Abscesses

The liver abscesses are caused by pyogenic (85 %), fungal (9 %), or amebic (6 %) agents and can present as multiple lesions up to 50 % of cases, with variable size between few millimeters and several centimeters. Classic pyogenic abscesses show rounded or oval morphology, with a thick hyperechoic wall, partially fluid content, with septa and sometimes gas and fluid levels in the context. CEUS allows better delineation of liver abscesses compared with conventional US, demonstrating more frequently peripheral enhancement around a central usually necrotic avascular area. Septa can be vascularized too, providing a peculiar " honeycomb" appearance [35].

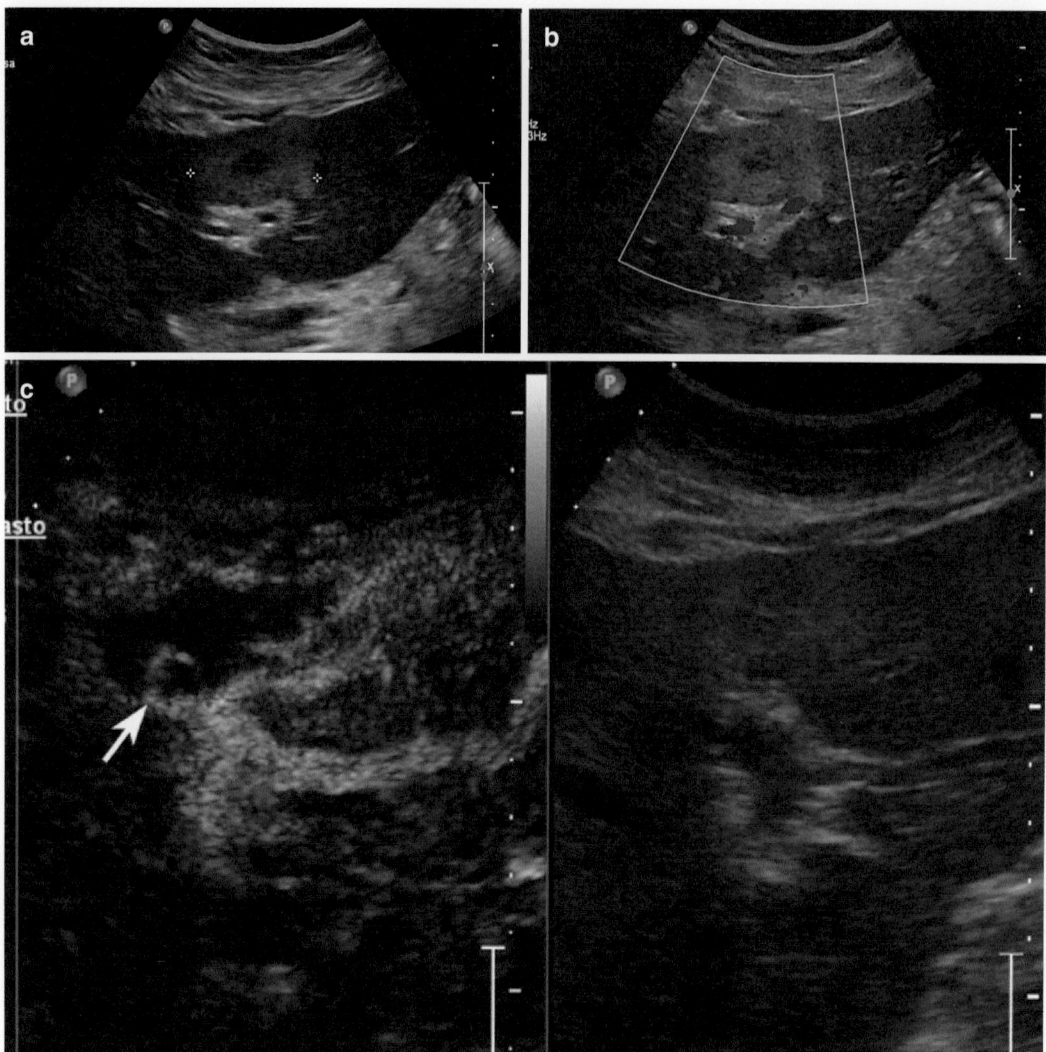

Fig. 2.19 Hepatic abscess in a 47-year-old woman with fever. (**a**) Central ascending subcostal baseline image reveals an inhomogeneous hyperechoic lesion with small central fluid area sized 4 cm in the IV hepatic segment (*calipers*) without any vascular signal at color-Doppler evaluation (**b**). At CEUS, the lesion shows substantially hypoechoic aspect with some thin enhancing septa in the arterial (**c**) and portal-venous (**d**) phases (*arrows*)

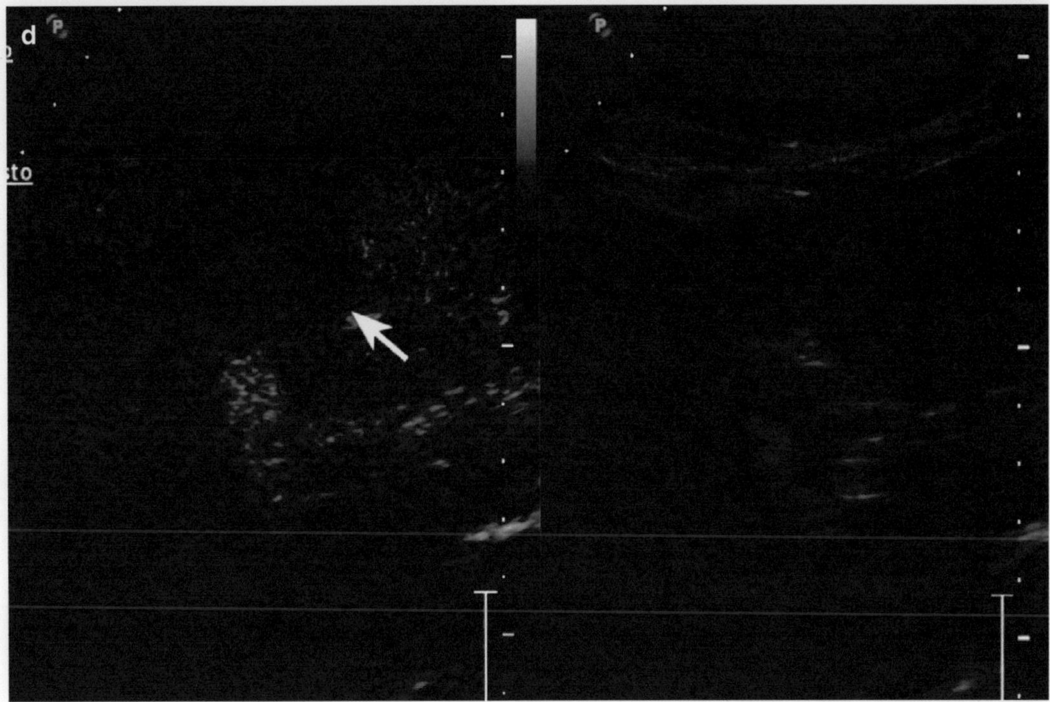

Fig. 2.19 (continued)

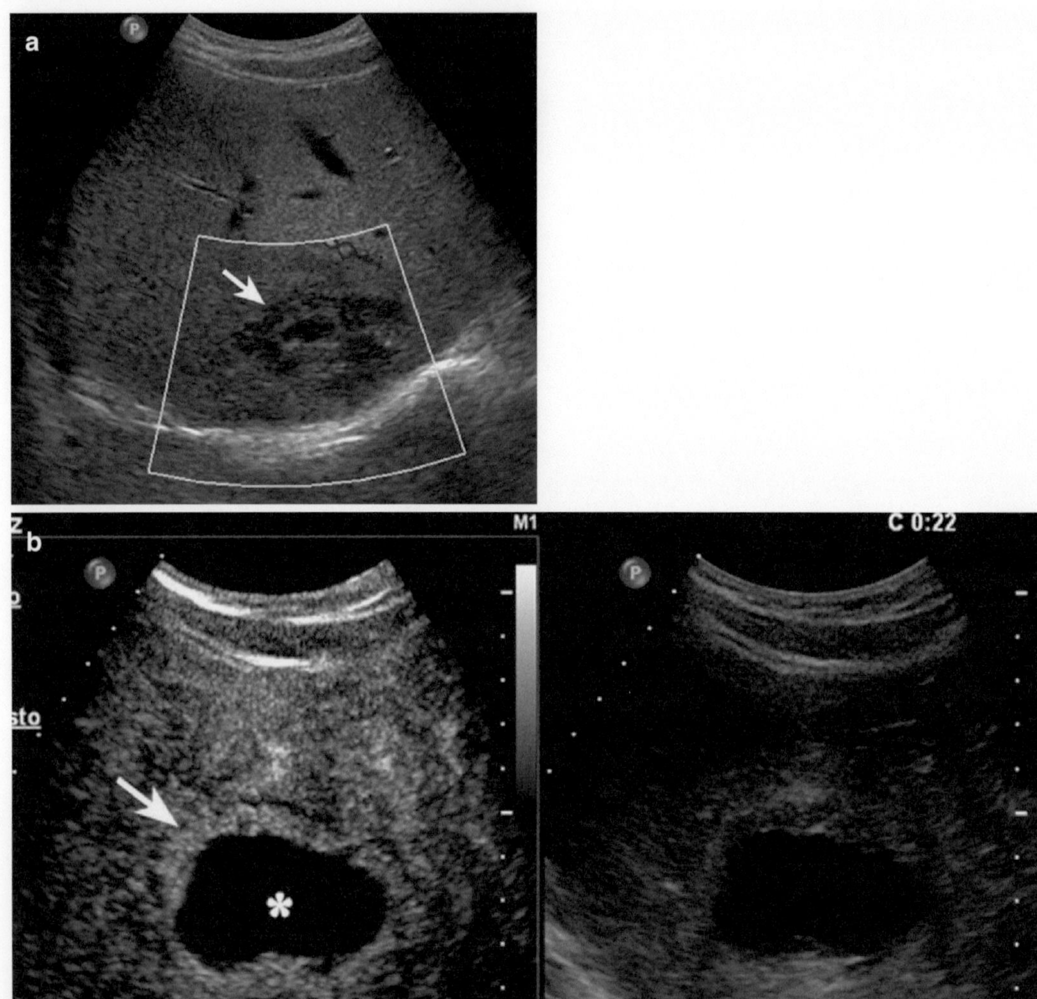

Fig. 2.20 Abscess in a 56-year-old woman with fever after biopsy. (**a**) Subcostal right baseline image reveals an inhomogeneous hypoechoic lesion sized 5.2 cm in the VII hepatic segment without any vascular signal at color-Doppler evaluation (*arrow*). (**b–d**) At CEUS, the lesions shows mainly peripheral enhancement surrounding a constantly hypoechoic area corresponding to the partly fluid collection (*asterisk*) throughout the vascular phases (*arrows*)

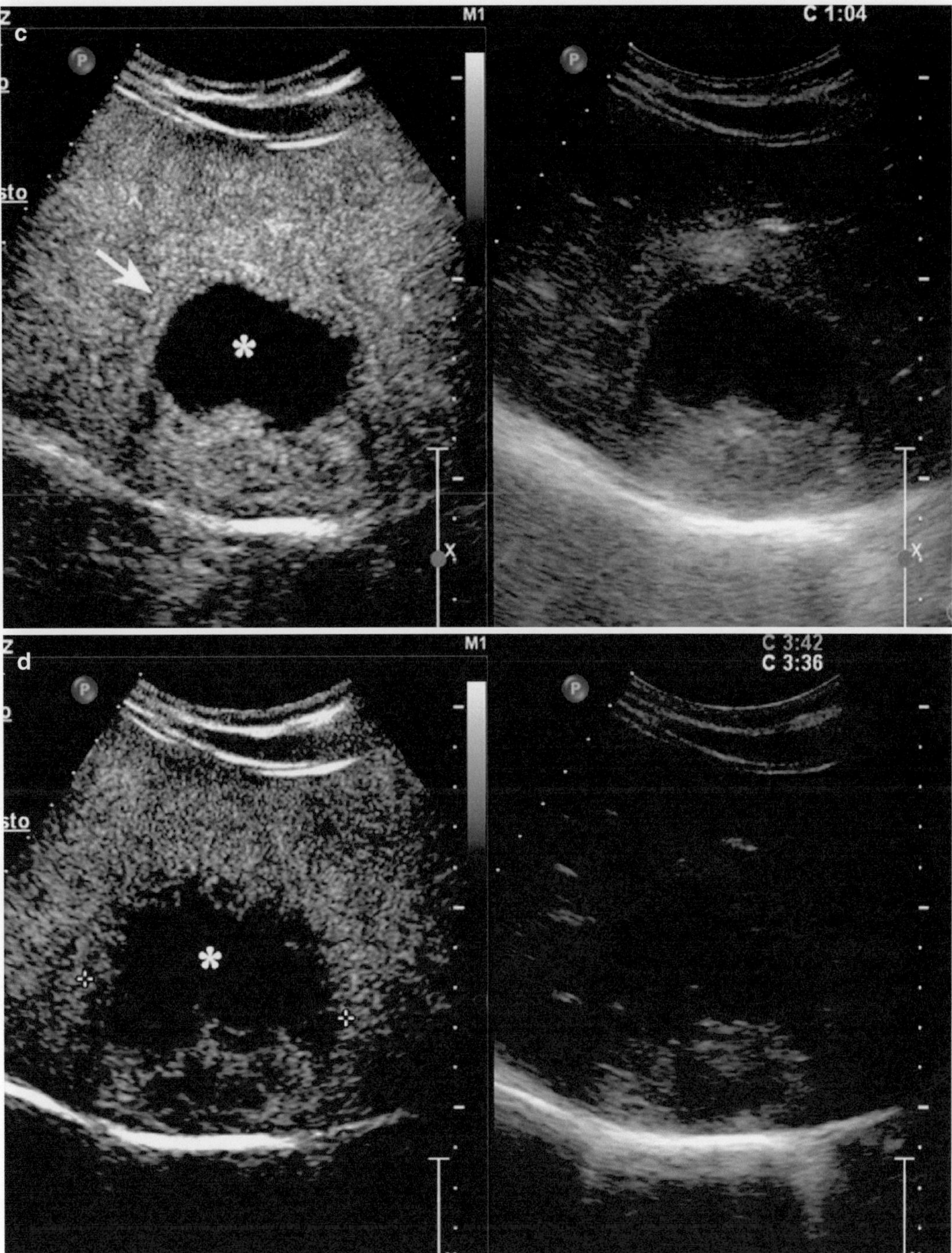

Fig. 2.20 (continued)

References

Hepatic Cysts

1. Ros PR, Menu Y, Vilgrain V et al (2001) Liver neoplasms and tumor-like conditions. Eur Radiol 11(Suppl 2):S145–S165
2. Nicolau C, Bru C (2004) Focal liver lesions: evaluation with contrast enhanced ultrasonography. Abdom Imaging 29:348–359

Hydatid Cyst

3. Nicolau C, Bru C (2004) Focal liver lesions: evaluation with contrast enhanced ultrasonography. Abdom Imaging 29:348–359
4. Antonopoulos P, Tavernaraki K, Charalampopoulos G et al (2008) Hydatid hepatic cysts rupture into the biliary tract, the peritoneal cavity, the thoracic cavity and the hepatic subcapsular space: specific computed tomography findings. Abdom Imaging 33(3):294–300

Hemangioma

5. Bartolotta TV, Midiri M, Quaia E et al (2005) Liver haemangiomas undetermined at gray-scale ultrasound: contrast-enhancement patterns with SonoVue and pulse-inversion US. Eur Radiol 15:685–693
6. Nicolau C, Catala V, Bru C (2003) Characterization of focal liver lesions with contrast-enhanced ultrasound. Eur Radiol 13(Suppl 3):70–78
7. Vilgrain V, Boulous L, Vullierme MP et al (2000) Imaging of atypical hemangiomas of the liver with pathological correlation. Radiographics 20:379–397
8. Kim TK, Choi BI, Han JK et al (2000) Hepatic tumors: contrast agent-enhancement patterns with pulse-inversion harmonic U.S. Radiology 216:411–417
9. Quaia E, Bertolotto M, Dalla Palma L (2002) Characterization of liver hemangiomas with pulse inversion harmonic imaging. Eur Radiol 12:537–544
10. Nino-Murcia M, Olcott EW, Jeffrey RB et al (2000) Focal liver lesions: pattern-based classification scheme for enhancement at arterial phase CT. Radiology 215:746–751
11. Quaia E, Bartolotta TV, Midiri M et al (2006) Analysis of different contrast enhancement patterns after microbubble-based contrast agent injection in liver hemangiomas with atypical appearance on baseline scan. Abdom Imaging 31:59–64
12. Bartolotta TV, Taibbi A, Galia M, Lo Re G, La Grutta L, Grassi R, Midiri M (2007) Centrifugal (inside-out) enhancement of liver hemangiomas: a possible atypical appearance on contrast-enhanced US. Eur J Radiol 64(3):447–455
13. Bartolotta TV, Midiri M, Galia M, Iovane A, Runza G, Carcione A, Lagalla R (2003) Atypical liver hemangiomas: contrast-enhancement patterns with SH U 508A and pulse-inversion US. Radiol Med 106(4):320–328
14. Bartolotta TV, Midiri M, Quaia E, Bertolotto M, Galia M, Cademartiri F, Lagalla R, Cardinale AE (2005) Benign focal liver lesions: spectrum of findings on SonoVue-enhanced pulse-inversion ultrasonography. Eur Radiol 15(8):1643–1649
15. Jang HJ, Kim TK, Burns PN, Wilson SR (2007) Enhancement patterns of hepatocellular carcinoma at contrast-enhanced US: comparison with histologic differentiation. Radiology 244:898–906
16. Dietrich CF, Sharma M, Gibson RN, Schreiber-Dietrich D, Jenssen C (2013) Fortuitously discovered liver lesions. World J Gastroenterol 19(21):3173–3188

Focal Nodular Hyperplasia

17. Anderson SW, Kruskal JB, Kane RA (2009) Benign hepatic tumors and iatrogenic pseudotumors. Radiographics 29:211–229
18. Prasad SR, Wang H, Rosas H et al (2005) Fat-containing lesions of the liver: radiologic-pathologic correlation. Radiographics 25:321–331
19. Herman P, Pugliese V, Machado MA et al (2000) Hepatic adenoma and focal nodular hyperplasia: differential diagnosis and treatment. World J Surg 24:372–376
20. Harvey CJ, Albrecht T (2001) Ultrasound of focal liver lesions. Eur Radiol 11:1578–1593
21. Bartolotta TV, Taibbi A, Midiri M et al (2010) Characterisation of focal liver lesions undetermined at grey-scale US: contrast-enhanced US versus 64-row MDCT and MRI with liver-specific contrast agent. Radiol Med 115:714–731
22. Ungermann L, Eliás P, Zizka J, Ryska P, Klzo L (2007) Focal nodular hyperplasia: spoke-wheel arterial pattern and other signs on dynamic contrast-enhanced ultrasonography. Eur J Radiol 63:290–294
23. Ronot M, Vilgrain V (2014) Imaging of benign hepatocellular lesions: current concepts and recent updates. Clin Res Hepatol Gastroenterol 38(6):681–688
24. Von Herbay A, Vogt C, Haussinger D (2002) Pulse inversion sonography in the early phase of the sonographic contrast agent Levovist: differentiation between benign and malignant focal liver lesions. J Ultrasound Med 21:1191–1200
25. Yen YH, Wang JH, Lu SN et al (2006) Contrast-enhanced ultrasonographic spoke-wheel sign in hepatic focal nodular hyperplasia. Eur J Radiol 60:439–444
26. Bartolotta TV, Taibbi A, Brancatelli G, Matranga D, Tumbarello M, Midiri M, Lagalla R (2014) Imaging findings of hepatic focal nodular hyperplasia in men and women: are they really different? Radiol Med 119(4):222–230

27. Bartolotta TV, Taibbi A, Matranga D, Malizia G, Lagalla R, Midiri M (2010) Hepatic focal nodular hyperplasia: contrast-enhanced ultrasound findings with emphasis on lesion size, depth and liver echogenicity. Eur Radiol 20(9):2248–2256

Hepatocellular Adenoma

28. Valls C, Iannacconne R, Alba E et al (2006) Fat in the liver: diagnosis and characterization. Eur Radiol 16(10):2292–2308
29. Prasad SR, Wang H, Rosas H et al (2005) Fat-containing lesions of the liver: radiologic-pathologic correlation. Radiographics 25(2):321–331
30. Herman P, Pugliese V, Machado MA et al (2000) Hepatic adenoma and focal nodular hyperplasia: differential diagnosis and treatment. World J Surg 24:372–376
31. Bartolotta TV, Taibbi A, Galia M et al (2007) Characterization of hypoechoic focal hepatic lesions in patients with fatty liver: diagnostic performance and confidence of contrast-enhanced ultrasound. Eur Radiol 17(3):650–661
32. Kim TK, Jang HJ, Burns PN et al (2008) Focal nodular hyperplasia and hepatic adenoma: differentiation with low-mechanical-index contrast-enhanced sonography. AJR Am J Roentgenol 190:58–66
33. Laumonier H, Cailliez H, Balabaud C, Possenti L, Zucman-Rossi J, Bioulac-Sage P, Trillaud H (2012) Role of contrast-enhanced sonography in differentiation of subtypes of hepatocellular adenoma: correlation with MRI findings. AJR Am J Roentgenol 199(2):341–348
34. Kim TK, Jang HJ, Burns PN, Murphy-Lavallee J, Wilson SR (2008) Focal nodular hyperplasia and hepatic adenoma: differentiation with low-mechanical-index contrast-enhanced sonography. AJR Am J Roentgenol 190:58–66

Abscesses

35. Liu GJ, Lu MD, Xie XY et al (2008) Real-time contrast-enhanced ultrasound imaging of infected focal liver lesions. J Ultrasound Med 27:657–666

3

3.1 Primary Malignant Tumor

3.1.1 Intrahepatic Cholangiocarcinoma

The intrahepatic cholangiocarcinoma (iCC) can present as single or multiple lesions tending to coalescence [1]. There are no wide study populations in literature about cholangiocarcinomas evaluated by means of CEUS, but according to reported data, the iCC presents inhomogeneous, mainly peripheral, contrast enhancement in the arterial phase with substantially hypovascular appearance in the extended portal-venous phase. The CEUS findings of ICC relate to the degree of neoplastic cell proliferation at pathological examination. Hyperenhancing areas in the tumor always indicated increased density of cancer cells. On the other side, fibrosis is more extended where hypovascular areas are detected [2]. Moreover, CEUS can definitely better delineate margins and evaluate more accurately the size and the possible involvement of the adjacent structures [3].

© Springer International Publishing Switzerland 2015
T.V. Bartolotta et al., *Atlas of Contrast-enhanced Sonography of Focal Liver Lesions*,
DOI 10.1007/978-3-319-17539-3_3

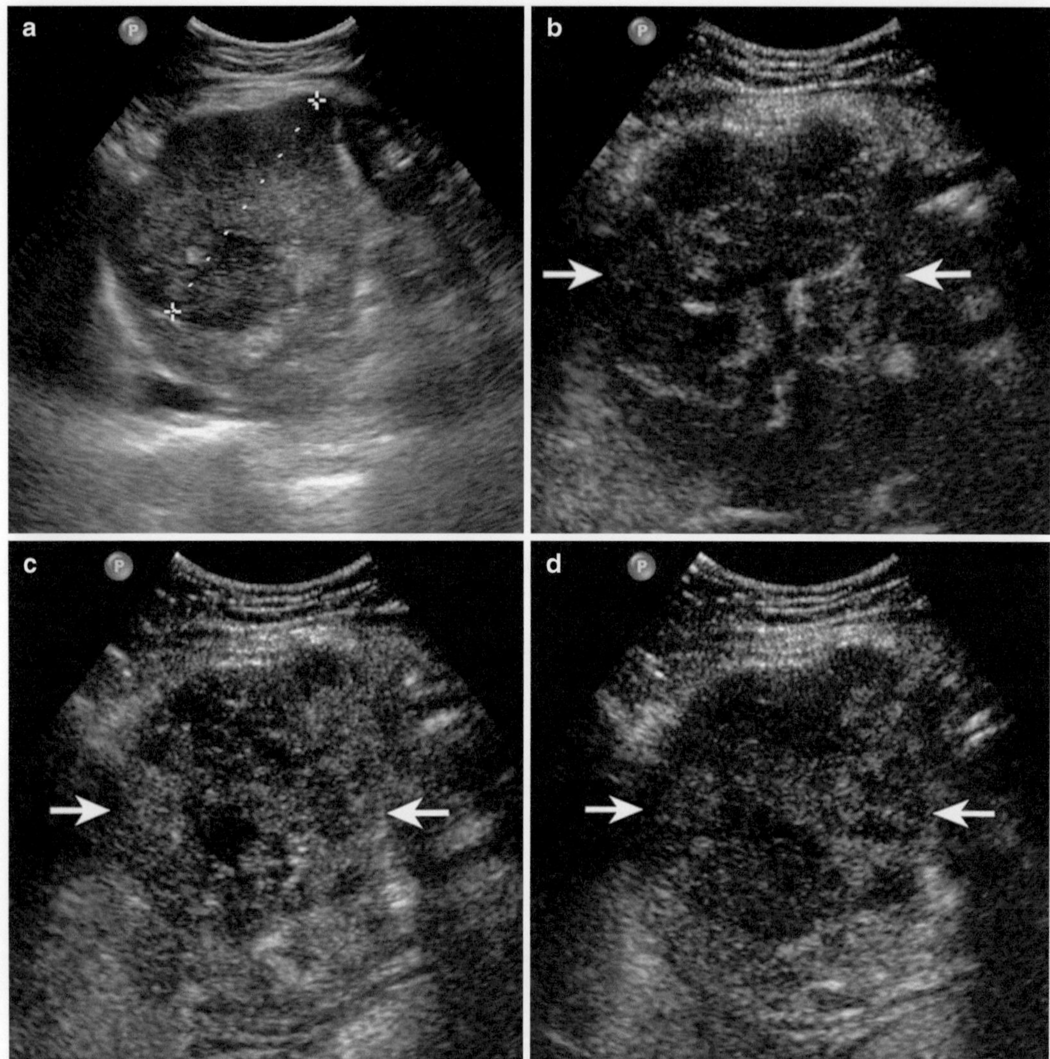

Fig. 3.1 Intrahepatic cholangiocarcinoma in a 62-year-old man. (**a**) Intercostal right baseline image reveals a large tumoral mass sized 8 cm in VI–VII hepatic segment (*calipers*). (**b**) At CEUS during the arterial phase, the lesion shows moderate and inhomogeneous enhancement (*arrows*). The lesion appears as hypoenhancing mass in comparison with adjacent parenchyma in the portal-venous (**c**) and late (**d**) phases (*arrows*)

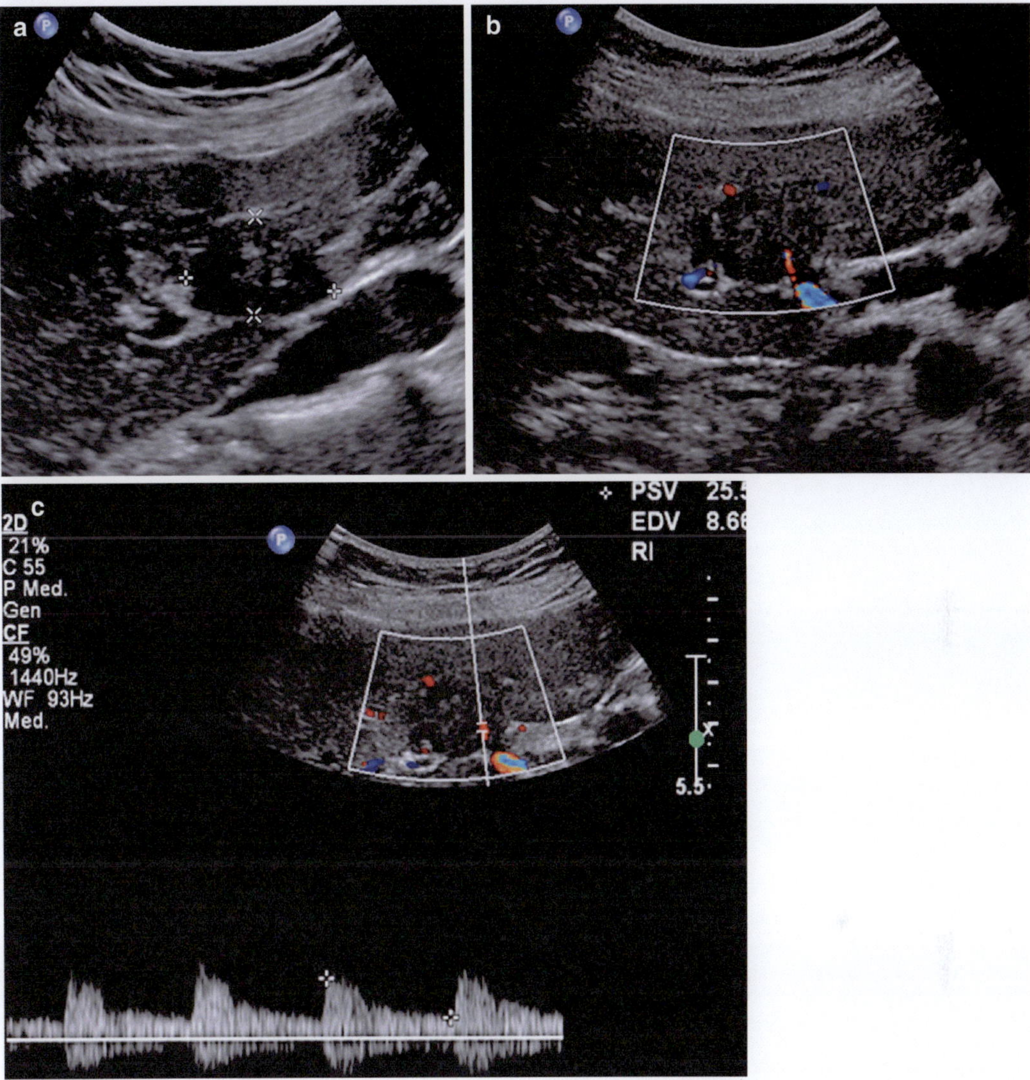

Fig. 3.2 Intrahepatic clear cell cholangiocarcinoma in a 65-year-old woman. (**a**) Baseline image reveals an inhomogeneous hypoechoic lesion sized 3.5 cm in V hepatic segment (*calipers*) with some arterial intralesional vessel at color-Doppler (**b**) and pulsed-Doppler (**c**) evaluation. (**d**) At CEUS during the arterial phase, the lesion is highly hypervascular with marked washout in the late phase (**e**) (*arrows*)

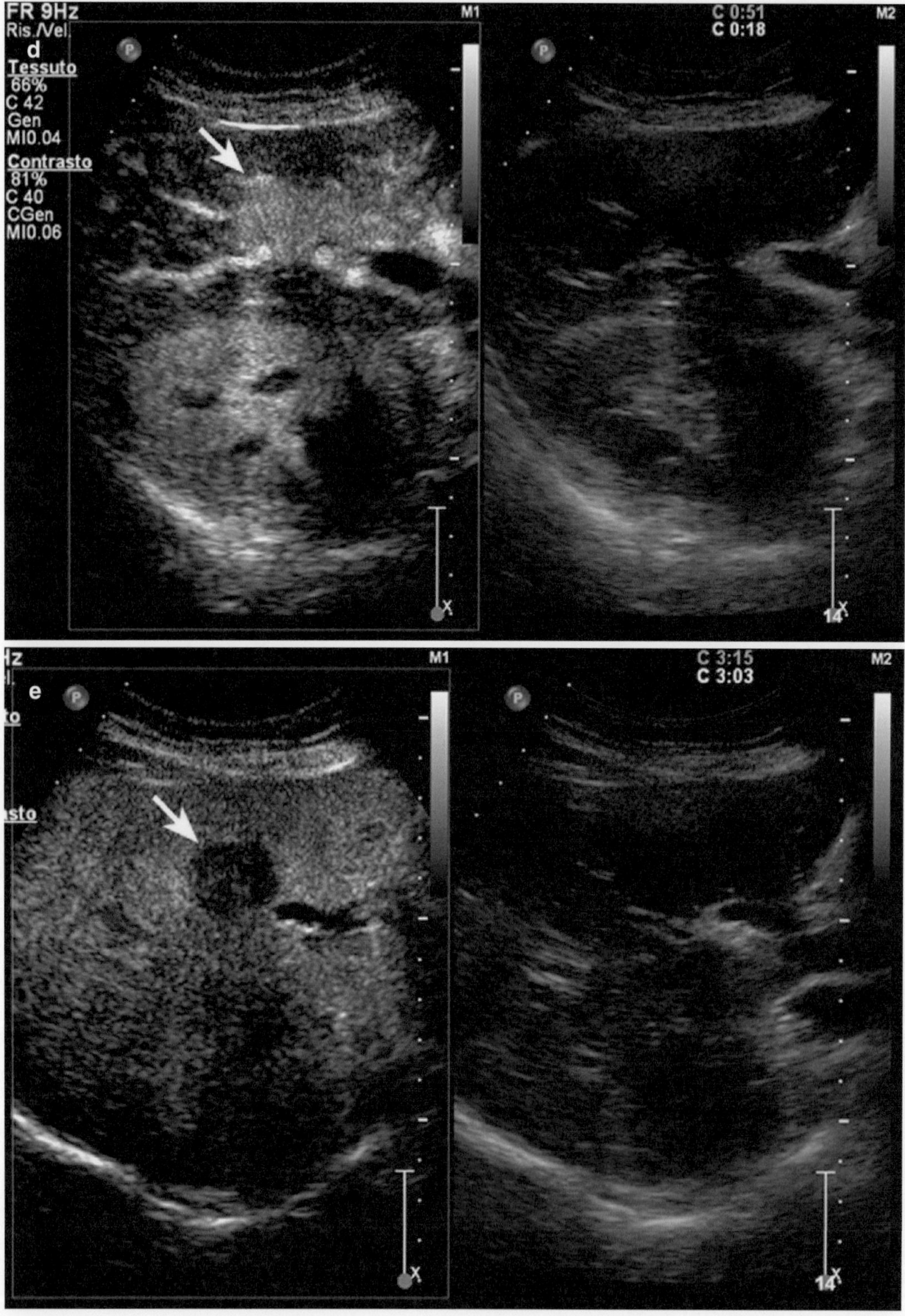

Fig. 3.2 (continued)

3.2 Cirrhotic Patients

Hepatocellular carcinoma (HCC) is the most common primary malignant liver neoplasm, more frequent in patients with HCV- and HBV-related cirrhosis, alcoholic cirrhosis, or hemochromatosis.

In the last 20 years, the incidence has risen sharply, so HCC represents the fifth most common cancer in the world and the third leading cause of death for neoplasm [4]. Except for the limited percentage of "de novo" HCC arising in noncirrhotic patients, the genesis of HCC is a "multistep" process including regenerating nodules and low- and high-grade dysplastic nodules up to overt HCC. During carcinogenesis process, liver vascularization becomes irregular and mostly arterial, with progressive reduced portal supply [5, 6]. Therefore, at CEUS, HCC occurs, in its typical form, as inhomogeneously hypervascular in the arterial phase, with more or less rapid washout in the extended portal-venous phase with hypoechoic appearance ("washout" sign) sometimes associated with a peripheral hypervascular halo (pseudocapsule) in the extended portal venous phase. However, according to the degree of differentiation, HCC may present different aspects. In fact, well-differentiated HCC, although hypervascular in the arterial phase, cannot be hypoechoic in the extended portal-venous phase causing misunderstanding at CEUS [7]. Moreover, CEUS allows the differentiation between HCC from regenerative and low-grade dysplastic nodules since these latter are not hypervascular in the arterial phase and are mainly indistinguishable from the remaining liver parenchyma in the extended portal-venous phase [8].

Being a real-time imaging modality, CEUS can be considered as problem-solving technique when CT or MR are not able to definitively characterize a nodule in cirrhotic patients allowing a better delineation of contrast enhancement behavior especially in the arterial phase when CT or MRI fails to show it because of incorrect arterial-phase timing [9, 10].

Nevertheless, CEUS has important limitations in surveillance programs of these patients because the short duration of the arterial phase does not allow to detect possible new hypervascular foci in all liver segments except with multiple contrast agent injections, but this is not feasible during daily clinical practice [11].

3.2.1   Regenerative Nodule

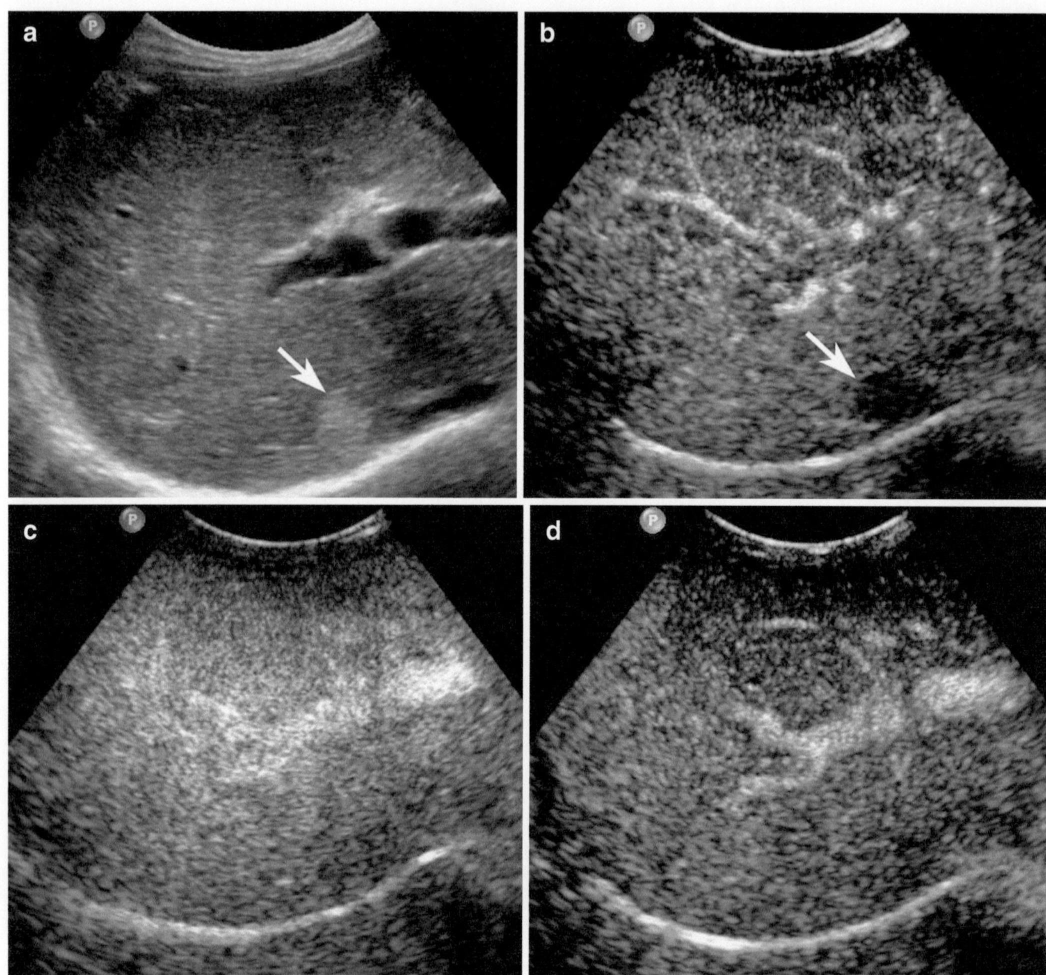

Fig. 3.3 Regenerative nodule in a 65-year-old man with liver cirrhosis. (**a**) Subcostal right baseline image reveals a well-defined hyperechoic lesion sized 2.1 cm in the VI–VII segment (*arrow*). (**b**) At CEUS during the arterial phase, the lesion shows no uptake of contrast agent (*arrow*). (**c**, **d**) The lesion appears isoechoic with respect to the surrounding liver parenchyma in the images acquired during the remaining vascular phases, revealing the same blood supply of the adjacent liver parenchyma

3.2.2 Dysplastic Nodule

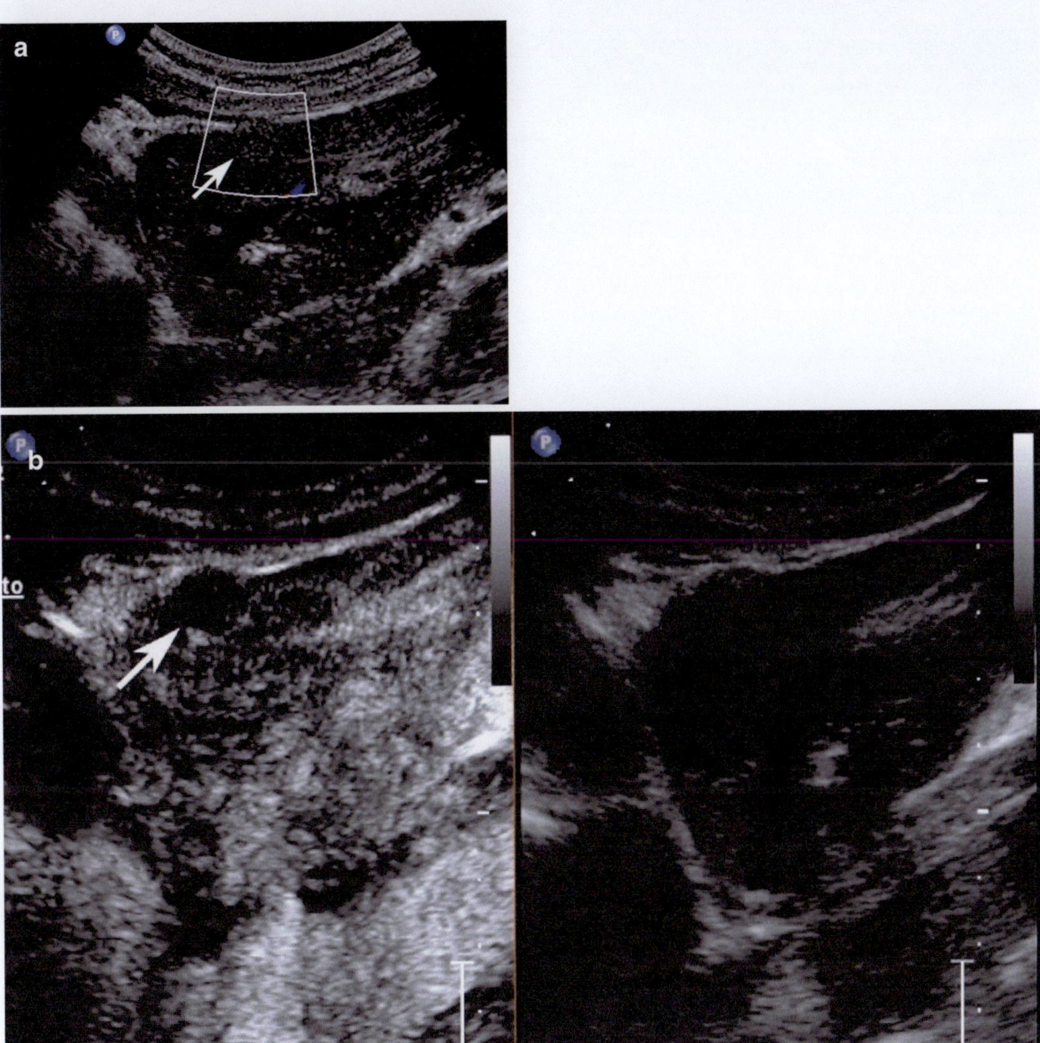

Fig. 3.4 Dysplastic nodule in a 58-year-old woman with HCV-related chronic hepatitis. (**a**) Sagittal subcostal baseline image reveals a moderately homogeneous partially exophytic hyperechoic nodule sized 1 cm in the left lobe without evident vascular signal at color-Doppler study (*arrow*). (**b–d**) At CEUS, the lesion presents hypoechoic aspect throughout the vascular study (*arrows*)

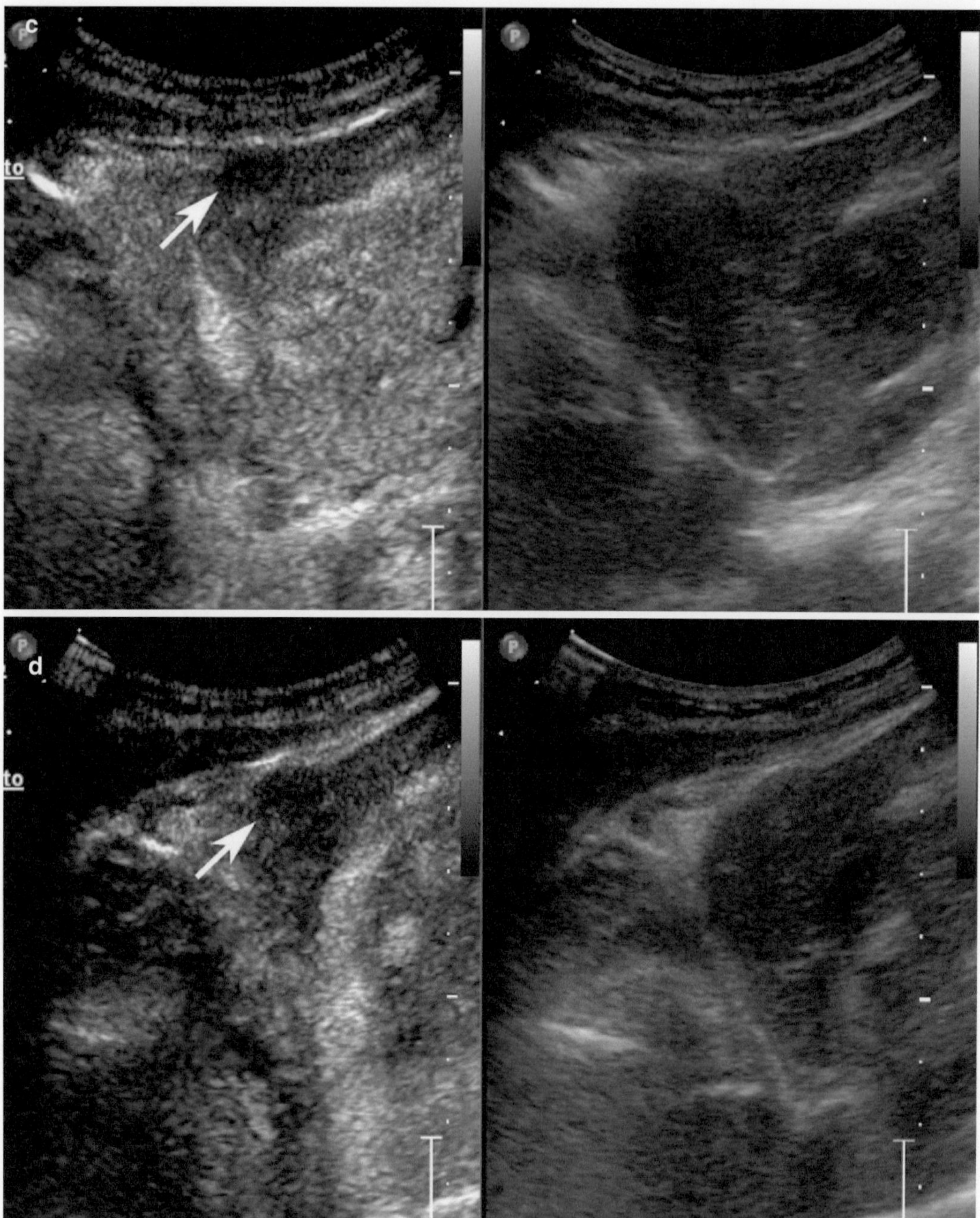

Fig. 3.4 (continued)

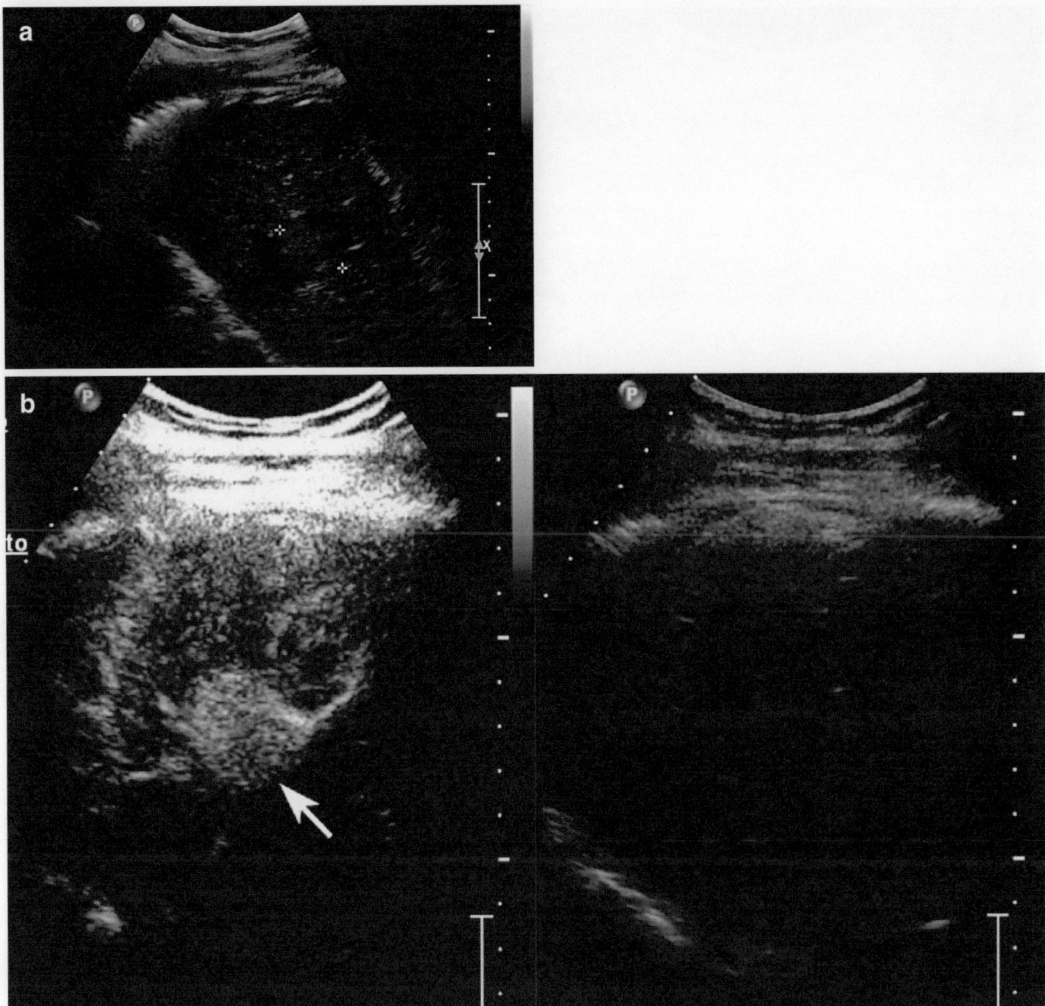

Fig. 3.5 Dysplastic nodule/early HCC in a 65-year-old-man with HCV-related chronic hepatitis. (**a**) Intercostal baseline image reveals an isoechoic lesion surrounded by a tiny hypoechoic rim sized 3 cm in the segment VIII (calipers). (**b**) At CEUS, the lesion presents a markedly hypervascular aspect in the arterial phase (*arrow*) becoming isovascular with respect to the surrounding liver parenchyma in the portal-venous (**c**) and late (**d**) phases (*arrows*)

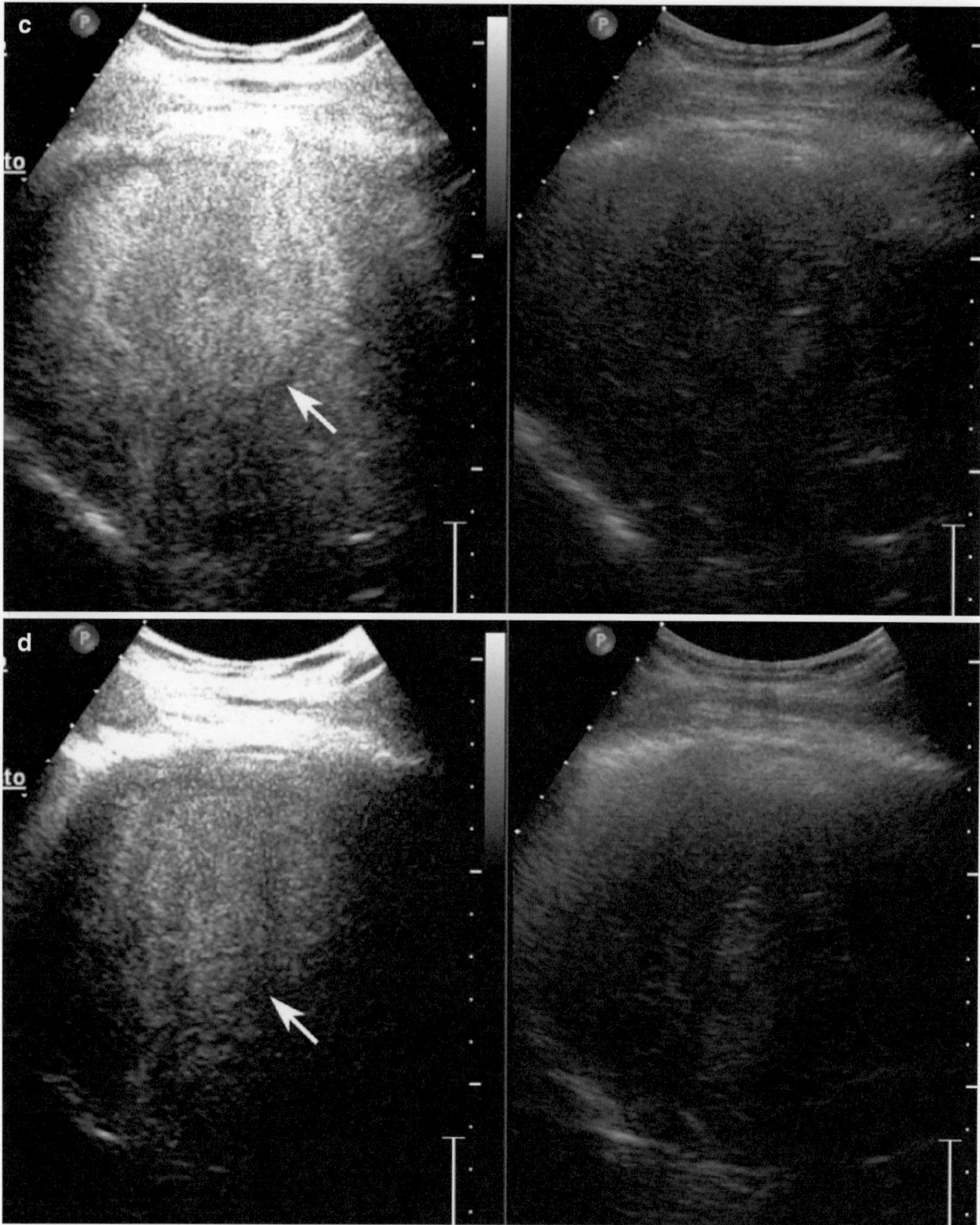

Fig. 3.5 (continued)

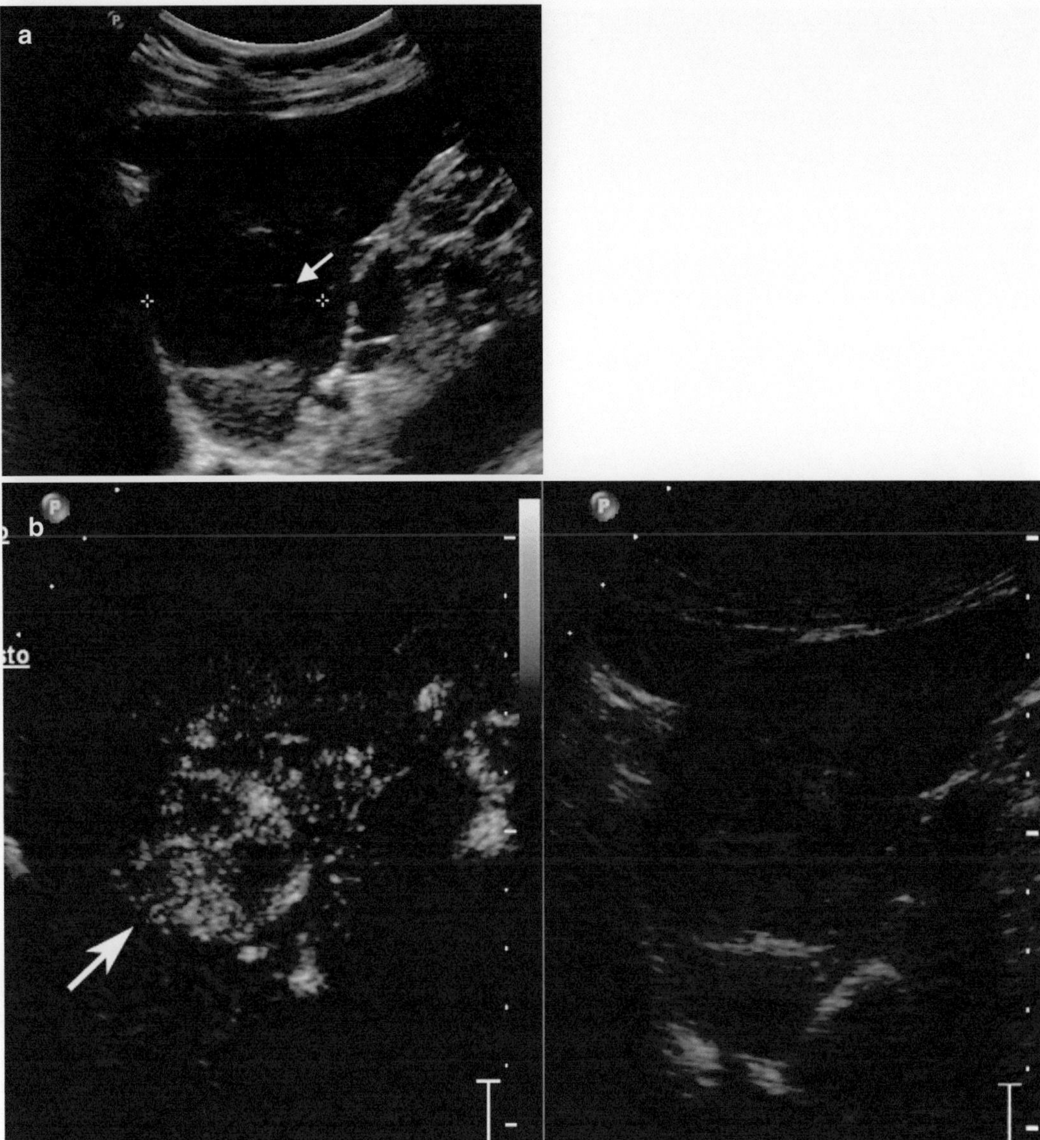

Fig. 3.6 Displastic nodule/early HCC in a 78-year-old man with HCV-related chronic hepatitis. (**a**) Sagittal subcostal baseline image reveals an inhomogeneous hypoechoic lesion sized 4.1 cm in the left lobe (*calipers*) with small fluid area in the context (*arrow*). (**b**) At CEUS, the lesion presents markedly hypervascular aspect in the arterial phase becoming isovascular with respect to the surrounding liver parenchyma in the portal-venous (**c**) and late (**d**) phases (*arrows*)

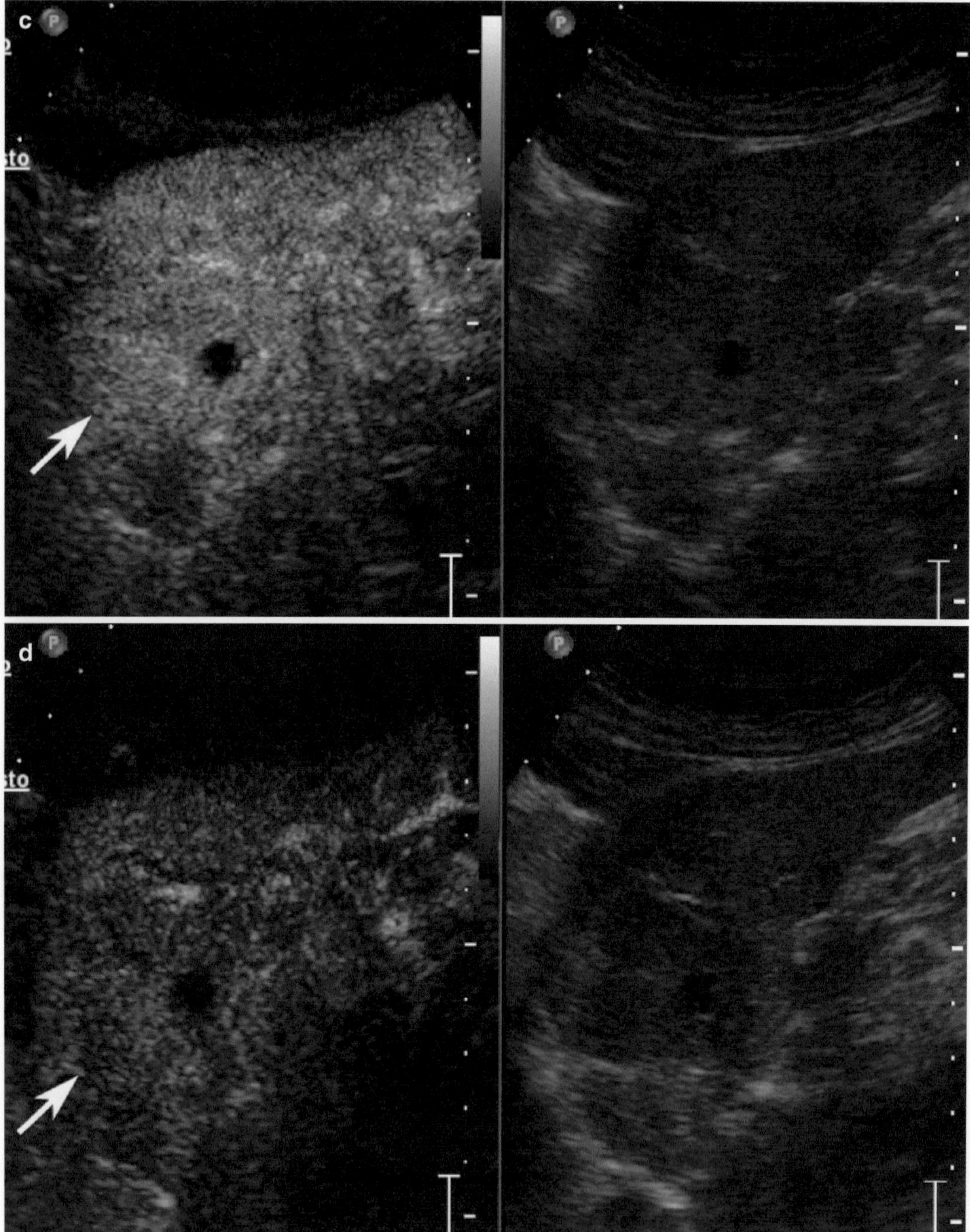

Fig. 3.6 (continued)

3.2.3 HCC

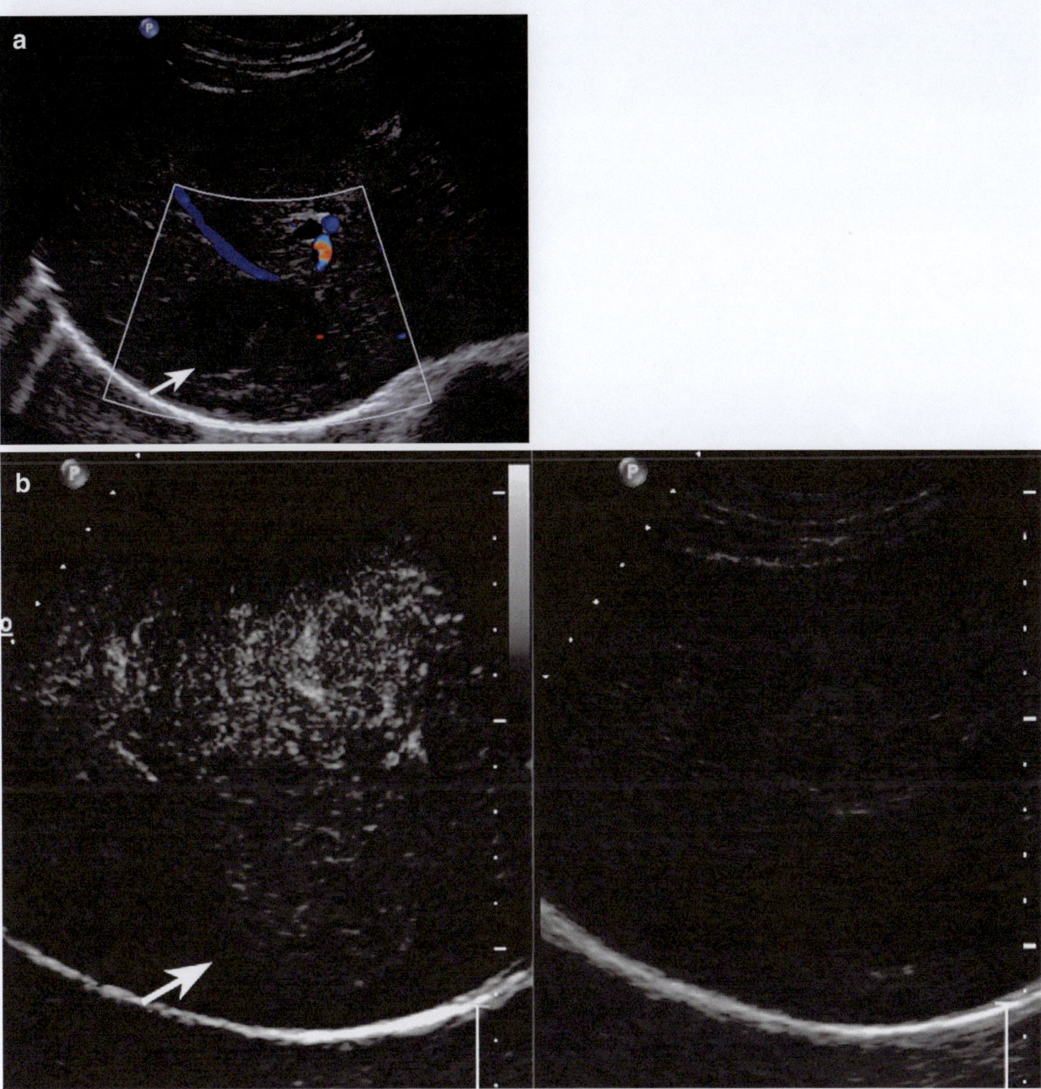

Fig. 3.7 HCC in a 78-year-old man with HCV-related chronic hepatitis. (**a**) Oblique ascending right subcostal baseline image reveals an inhomogeneous hypoechoic lesion sized 4.5 cm in the VII hepatic segment with tiny peripheral vascular signal at color-Doppler evaluation (*arrow*). (**b**) At CEUS, the lesion presents moderately hypervascular aspect in the arterial phase followed by washout in the extended portal-venous phase (**c**) (*arrows*)

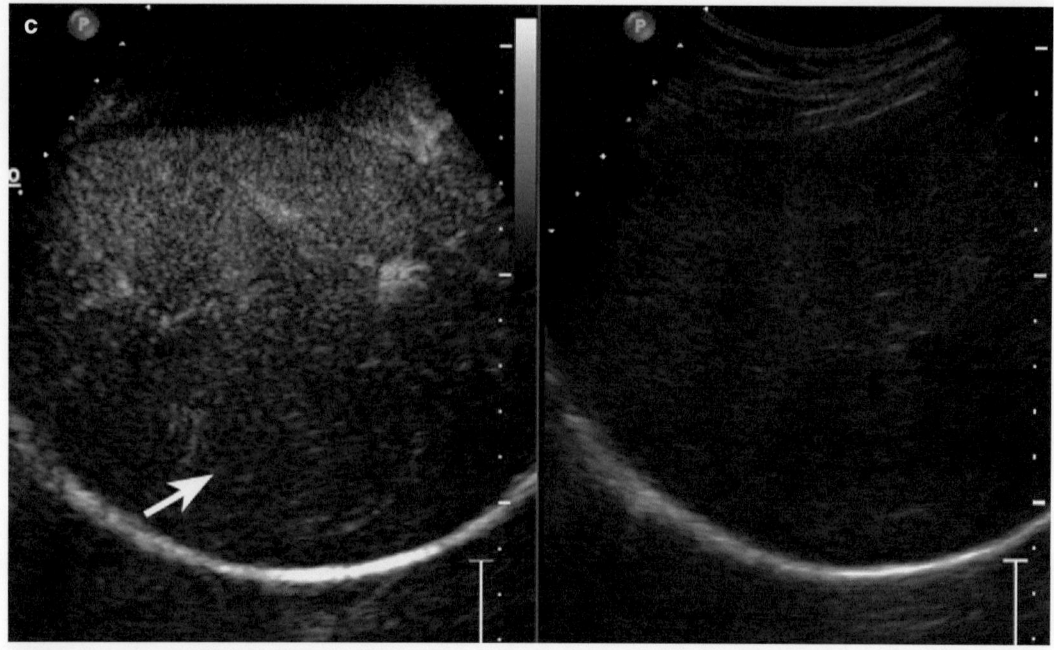

Fig. 3.7 (continued)

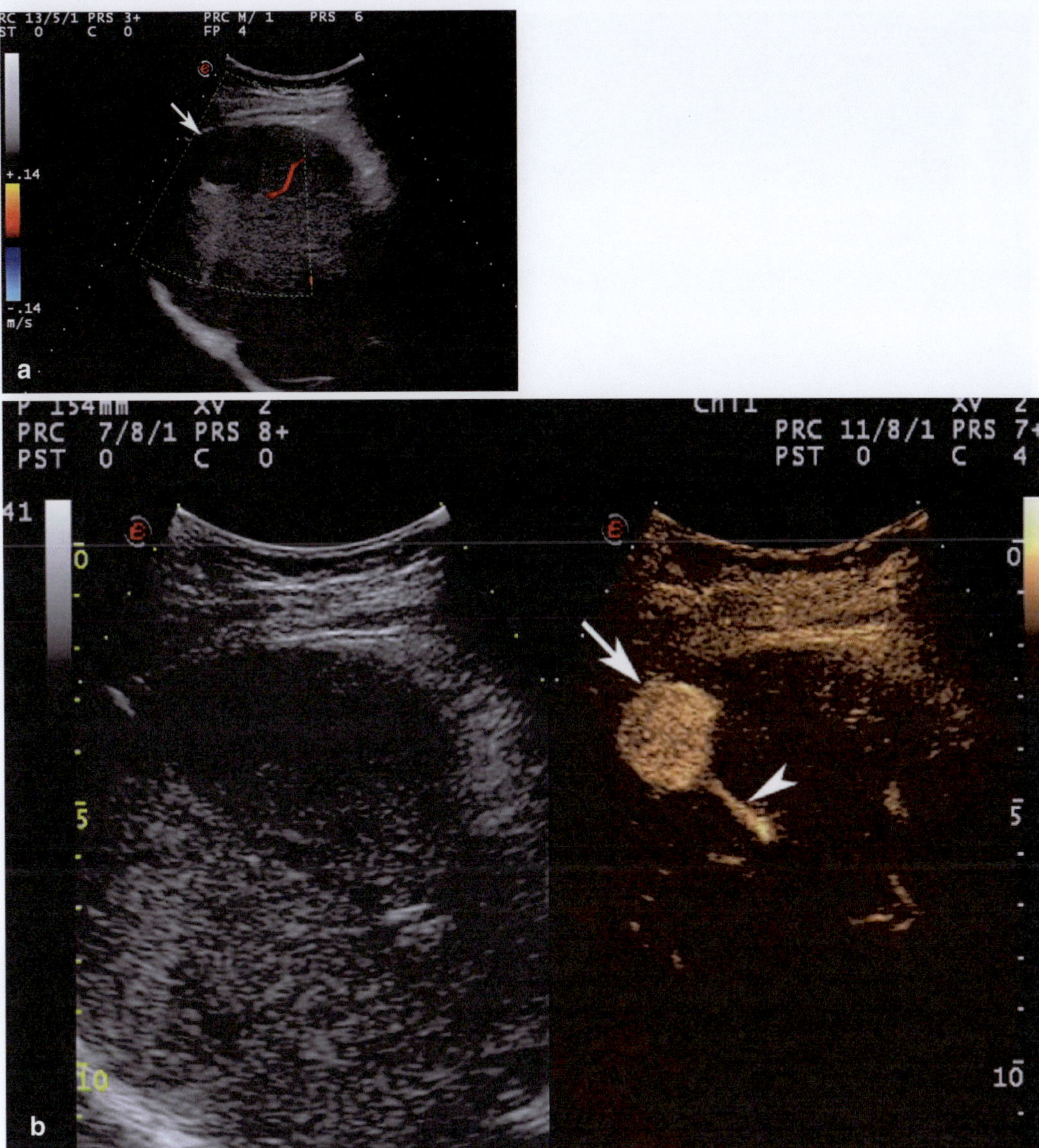

Fig. 3.8 HCC in a 64-year-old woman with HCV-related chronic hepatitis. (**a**) Intercostal right baseline US image reveals a homogeneous markedly hypoechoic lesion sized 3.2 cm in the VIII hepatic segment without vascular signal at color-Doppler evaluation (*arrow*). (**b**) At CEUS, the lesion shows a strong contrast enhancement (*arrow*) with evident feeding vessel (*arrowhead*) in the arterial phase. The lesion is not evident in the portal-venous phase (**c**) but shows a clear-cut washout in the late phase (**d**) (*arrow*)

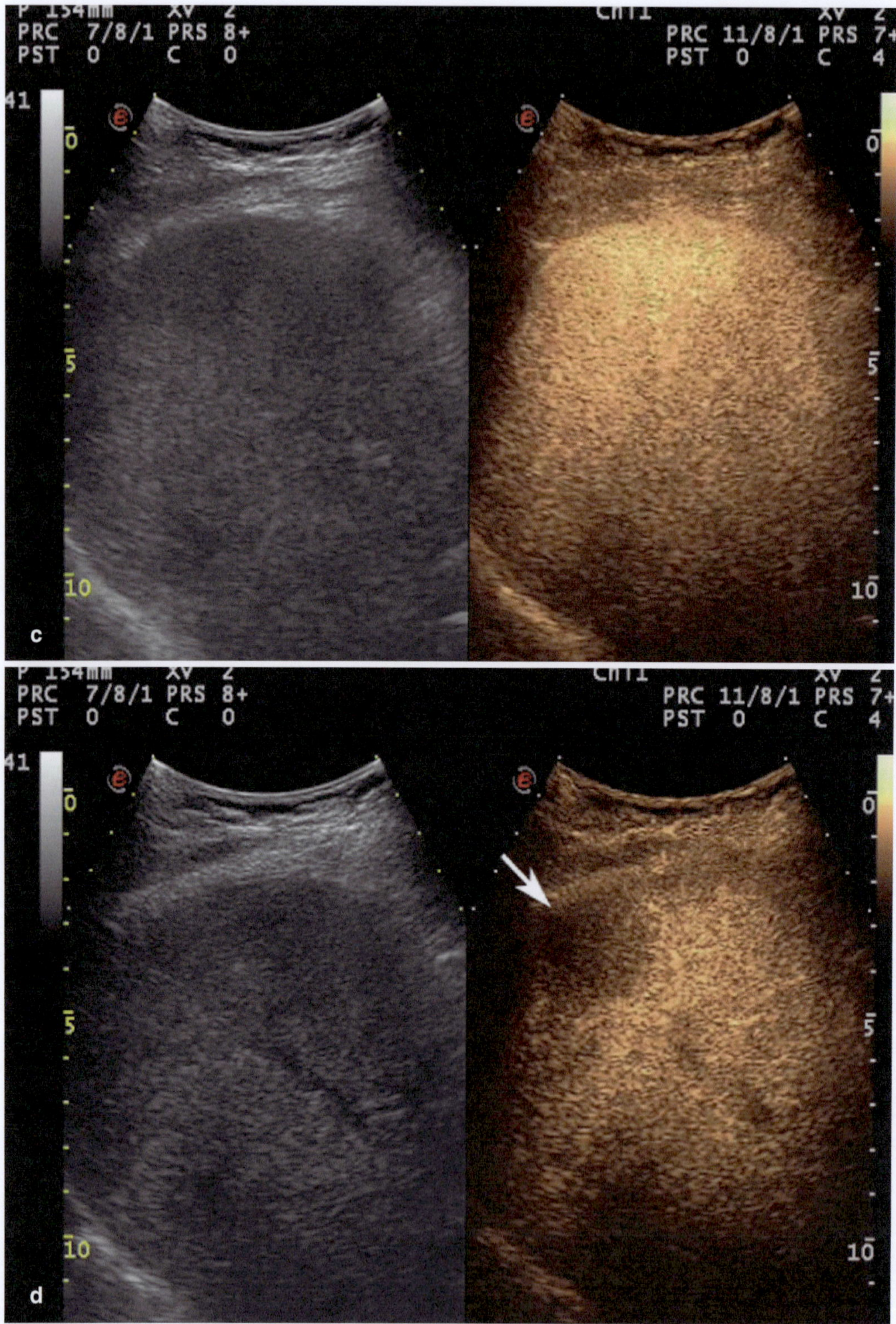

Fig. 3.8 (continued)

3.3 Metastases

The detection of liver metastases is of utmost importance either for the choice of the most adequate therapy and during the follow-up or also in consideration of several available treatment options [12]. For this purpose, the sensitivity of conventional US is, in spite of its wide employment, much lower (40–77 %) than that reported for CT or MRI, dropping below 20 % for lesions ≤1 cm [13].

On the other hand, several studies showed high diagnostic accuracy of CEUS with respect to conventional US both in the detection and characterization of liver metastases with a significant increase in the total number of identified lesions in patients with already known or suspected metastases adequately explorable at US [14, 15].

In fact, thanks to the newest technologies, CEUS reached values of sensitivity and specificity similar to CT and MR, respectively, 80–95 % and 84–98 % [16].

CEUS is particularly useful in the detection of lesions <1 cm or isoechoic with respect to the surrounding liver parenchyma and, therefore, not detectable at conventional US [17].

Grayscale US appearance of liver metastases is variable, and both color- or power-Doppler are not helpful because the majority of the metastases do not present macrovessels. On the contrary, CEUS is highly reliable in the detection of neo-angiogenesis phenomenon occurring within liver metastases. So the metastases show different aspects in the arterial phase at CEUS. They can present a peripheral ring of contrast enhancement, a "dotted" aspect with some tiny hyperechoic spots in the context, or a hyper- or hypovascular appearance. Anyway, they always have to show a hypovascular aspect during the extended portal-venous phase ("washout" sign) and appear hypoechoic [18].

3.3.1   Hypervascular Metastases

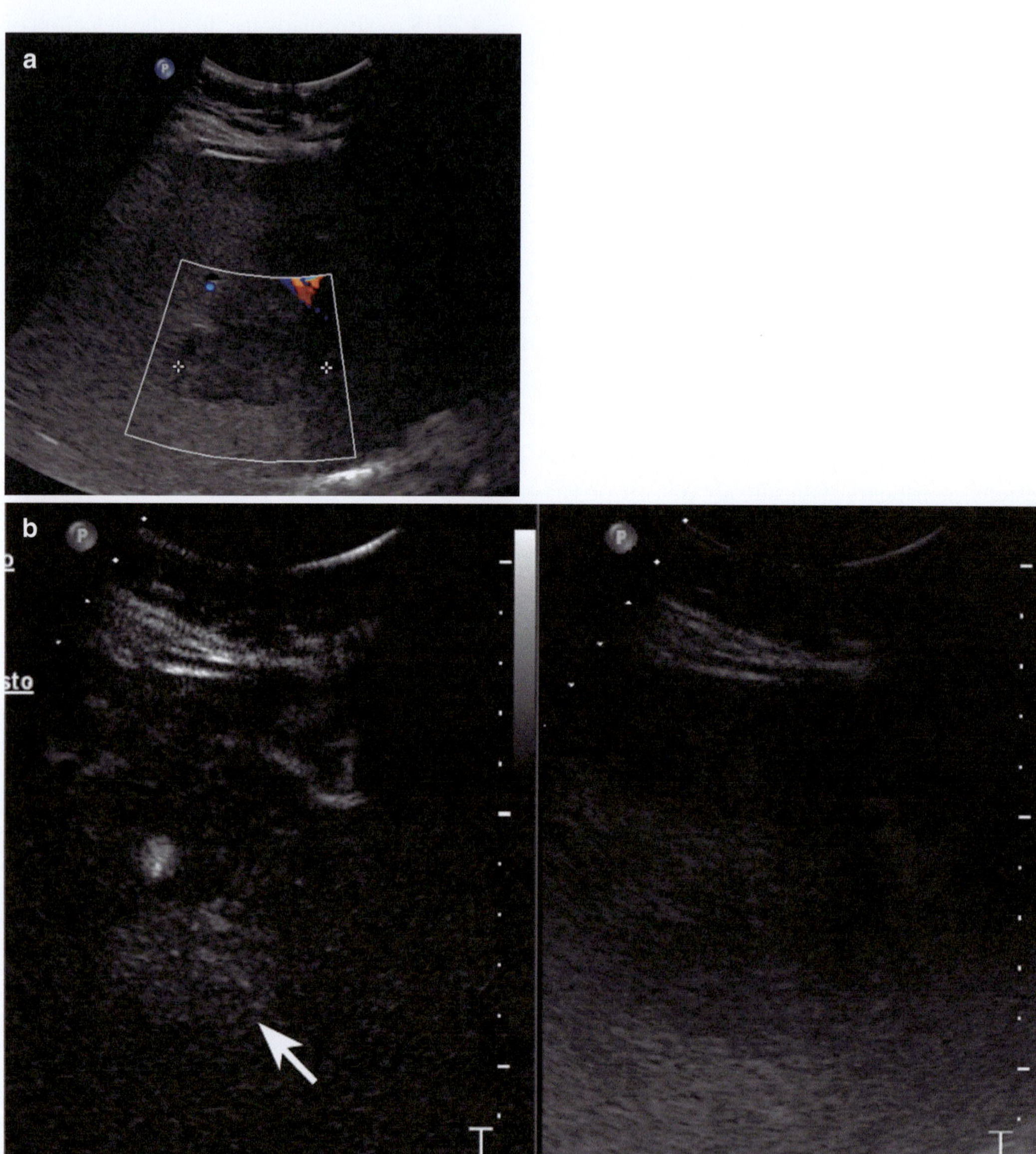

Fig. 3.9 Liver metastasis from renal cell carcinoma in a 52-year-old woman. (**a**) Oblique ascending right subcostal baseline US image reveals a well-defined hypoechoic lesion sized 4.9 cm in the VIII hepatic segment without evident vascularization at color-Doppler evaluation (calipers). (**b**) The lesion shows an intense and homogeneous contrast enhancement in the late arterial phase (*arrow*). In the portal-venous (**c**) and late (**d**) phases, it shows progressive washout and appears hypoechoic with respect to the surrounding liver parenchyma, suggesting malignancy (*arrows*)

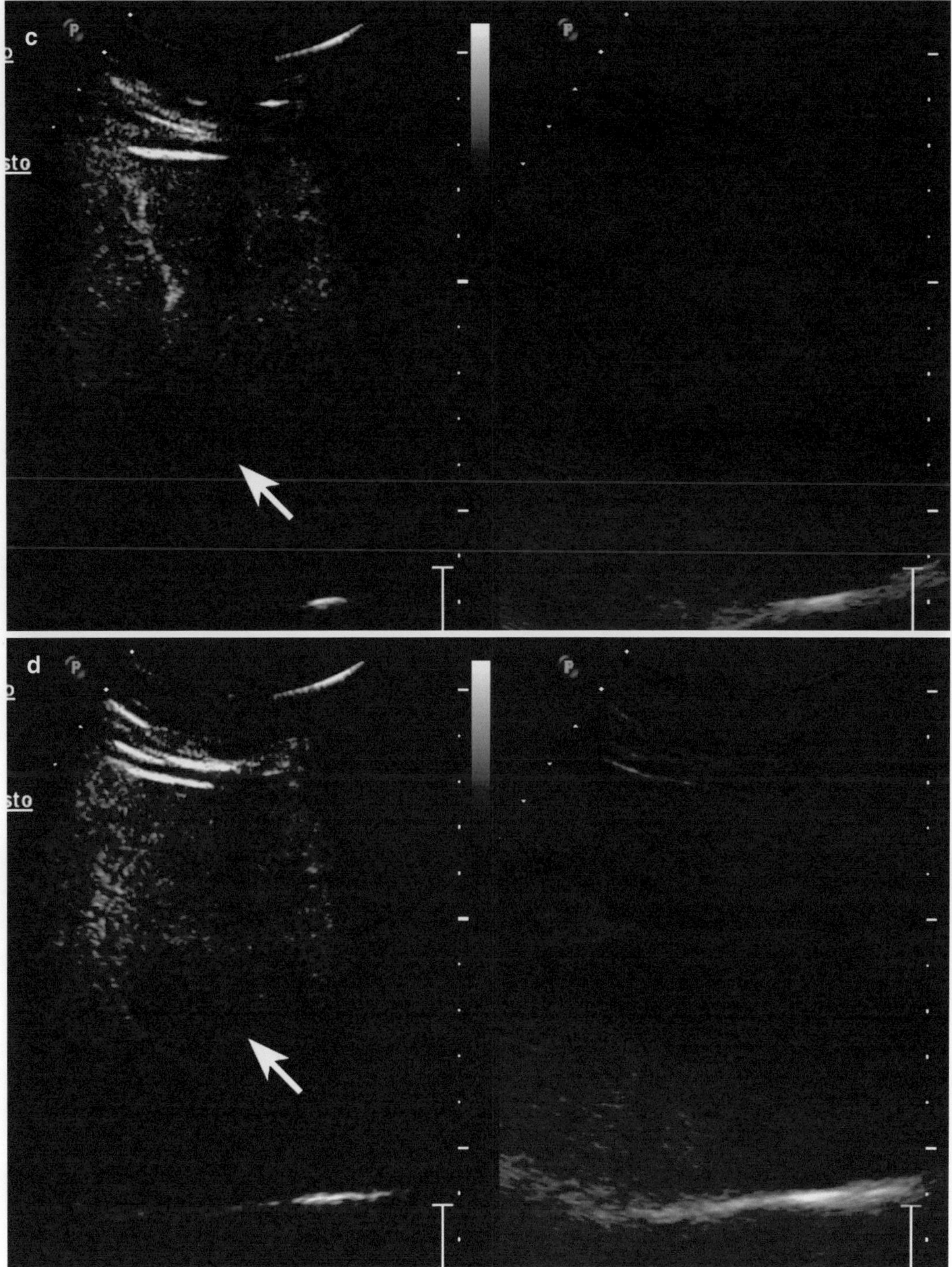

Fig. 3.9 (continued)

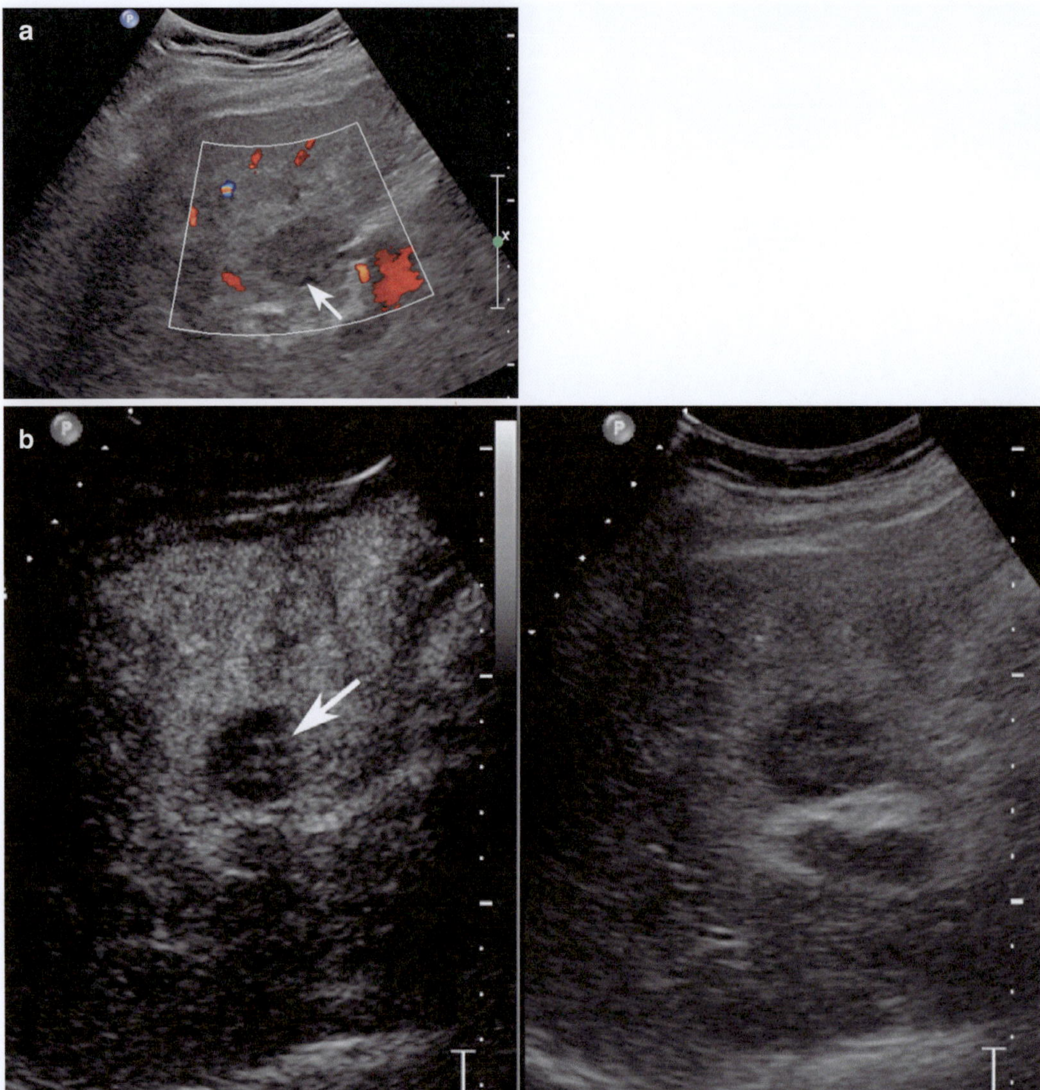

Fig. 3.10 Liver metastasis from small bowel adenocarcinoma in a 72-year-old man. (**a**) Oblique ascending right subcostal US image reveals a well-defined hypoechoic lesion sized 2.8 cm in the IV hepatic segment without evident vascular signal (*arrow*). (**b**) On the image obtained in the arterial phase, tiny hypervascular spots are evident within the lesion (*dotted aspect*) (*arrow*). In the portal-venous (**c**) and late (**d**) phases, it shows a marked hypoechoic aspect with respect to the surrounding liver parenchyma (*arrows*)

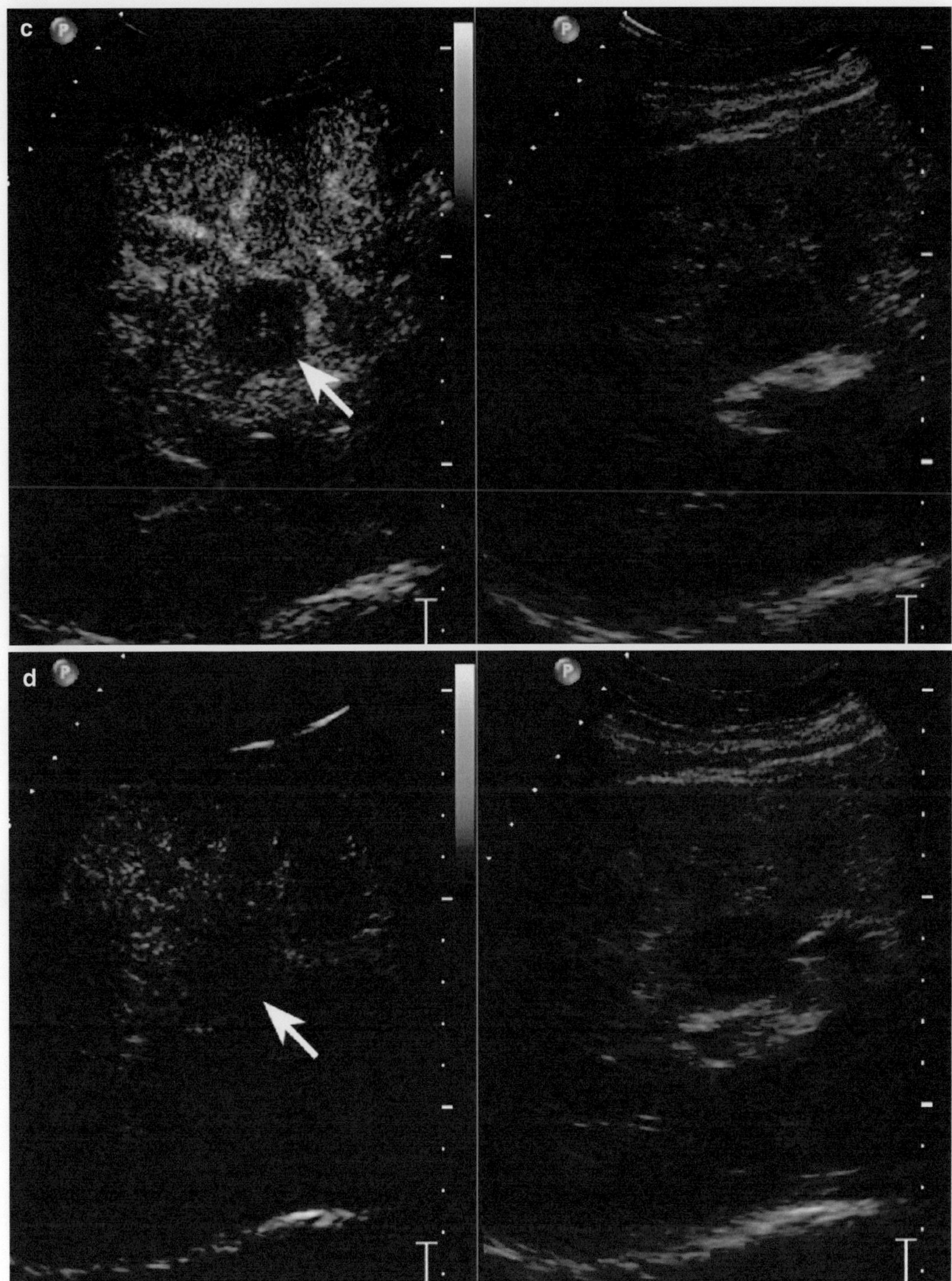

Fig. 3.10 (continued)

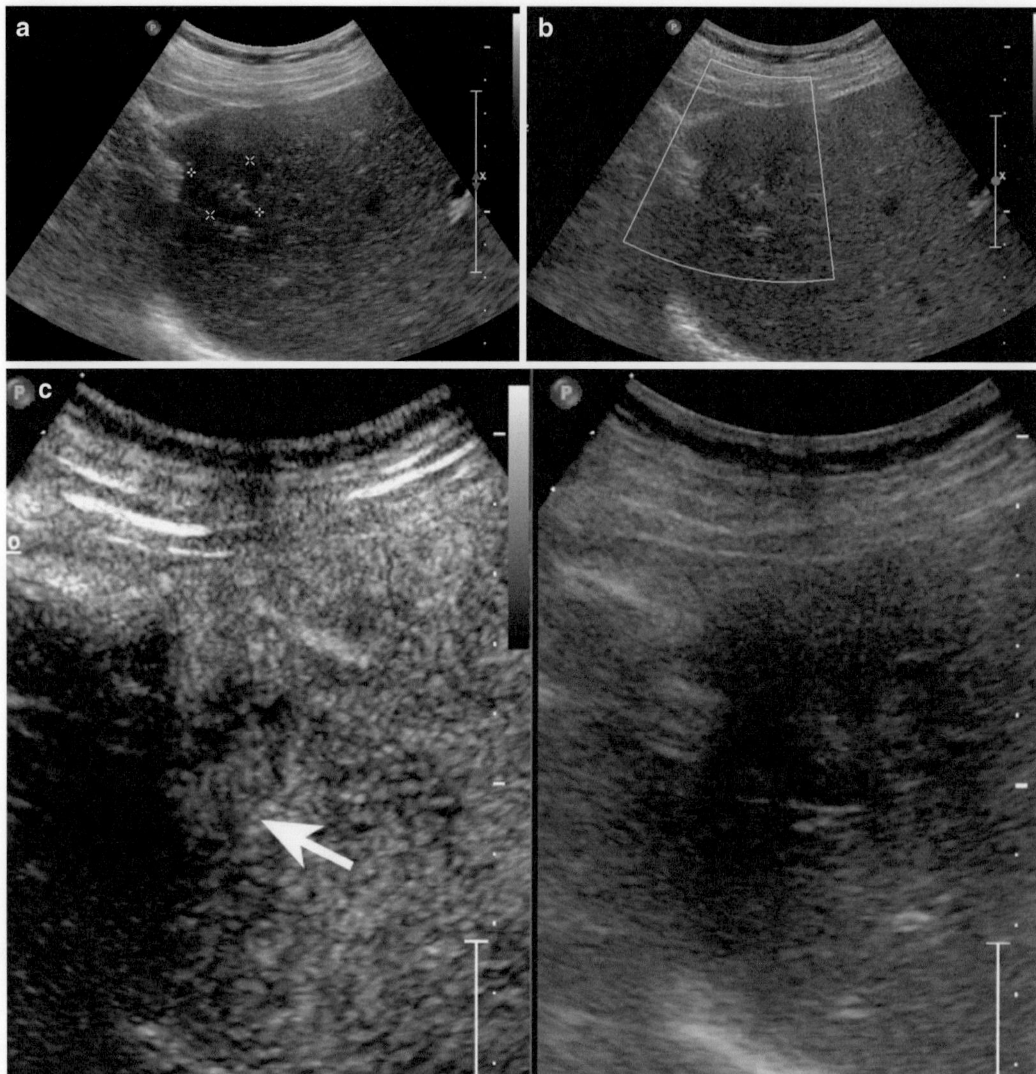

Fig. 3.11 Liver metastasis from lung cancer in a 78 year-old-woman. (**a**) Oblique ascending right subcostal baseline image in a 67-year-old woman shows a 2.4 mm-sized inhomogeneous lesion located in the VII hepatic segment (calipers). (**b**) At color-Doppler, no vascular signal is evident. (**c**) At CEUS, the lesion presents moderate and inhomogeneous contrast enhancement in the arterial phase showing a clear-cut washout in the extended portal-venous phase (**d**) (*arrows*)

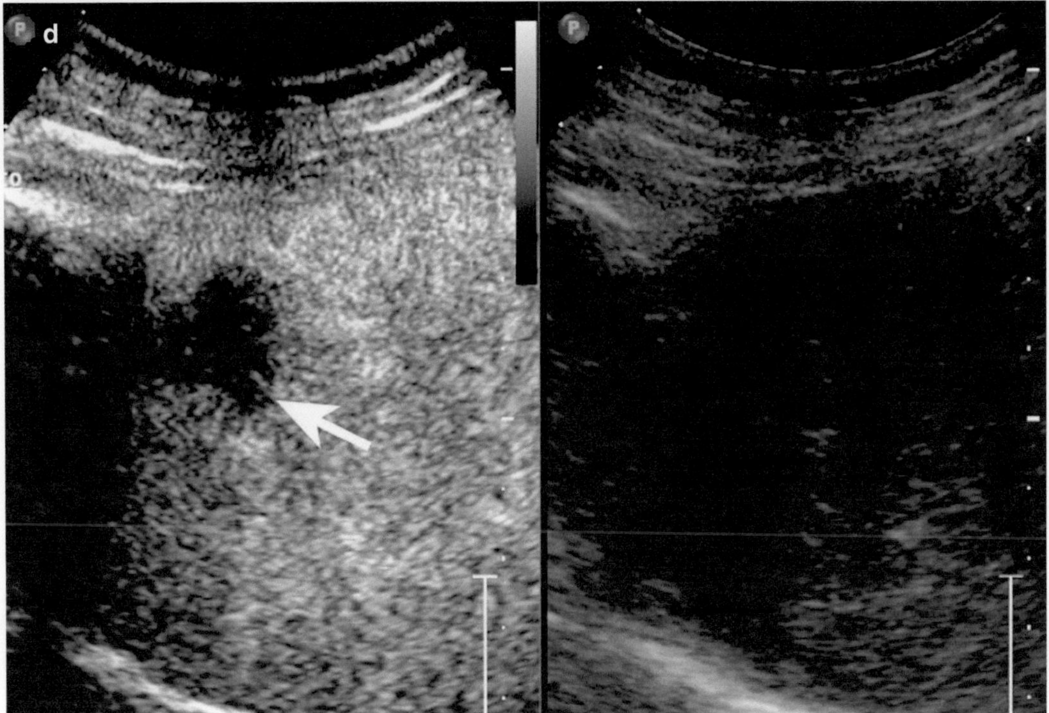

Fig. 3.11 (continued)

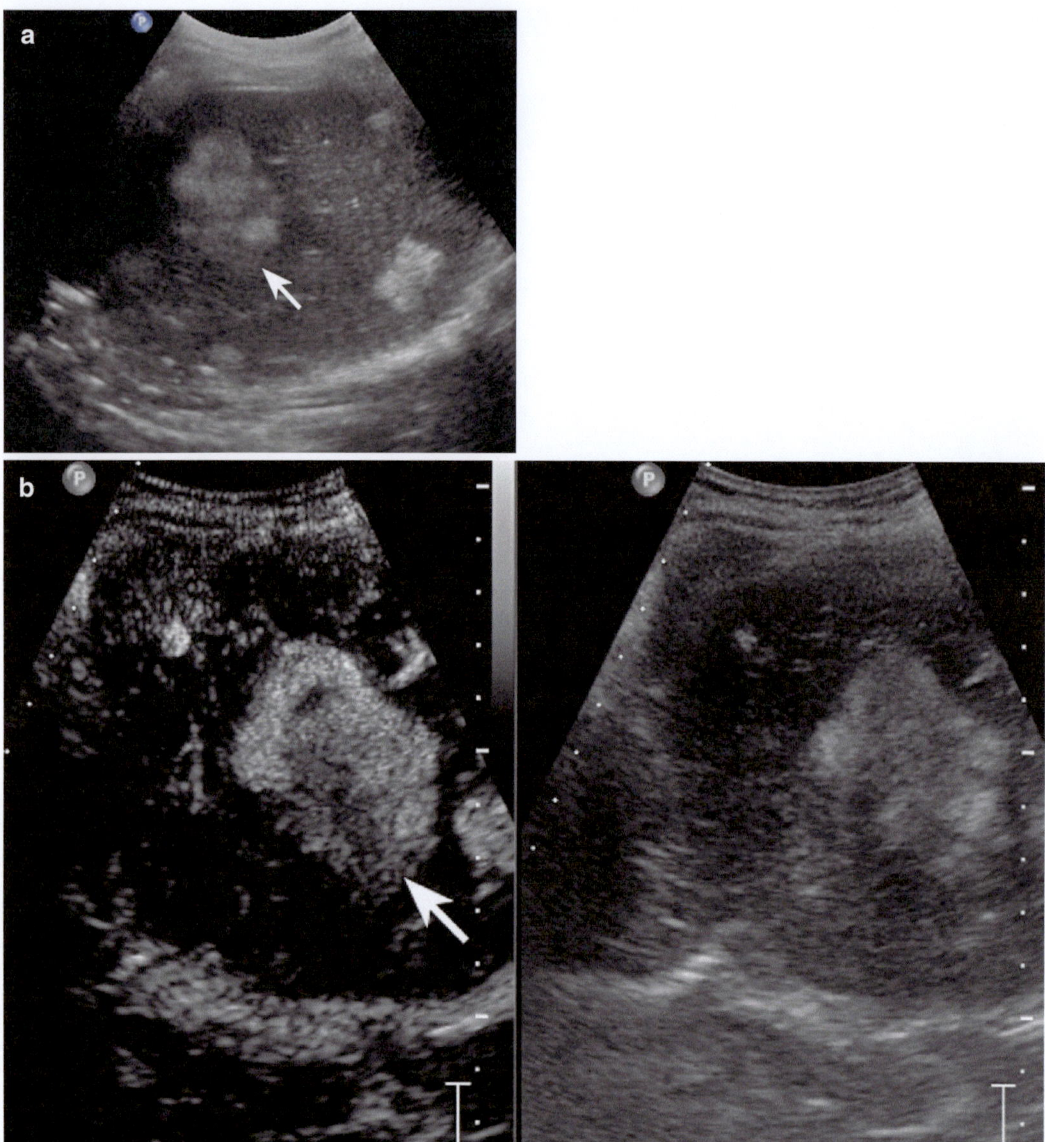

Fig. 3.12 Multiple liver metastasis from mucinous colorectal carcinoma in a 67-year-old woman. (**a**) Oblique ascending right subcostal baseline image reveals a well-defined hyperechoic lesion with lobulated margins sized 4.8 cm in the VII–VIII hepatic segment (*arrow*). (**b**) On the image obtained in the arterial phase, the lesion shows a clear-cut quite homogeneous contrast enhancement (*arrow*). In the portal-venous (**c**) and late (**d**) phases, it shows a clear-cut washout and appears hypoechoic with respect to the surrounding liver parenchyma surrounded by a peripheral hypervascular rim (*arrows*)

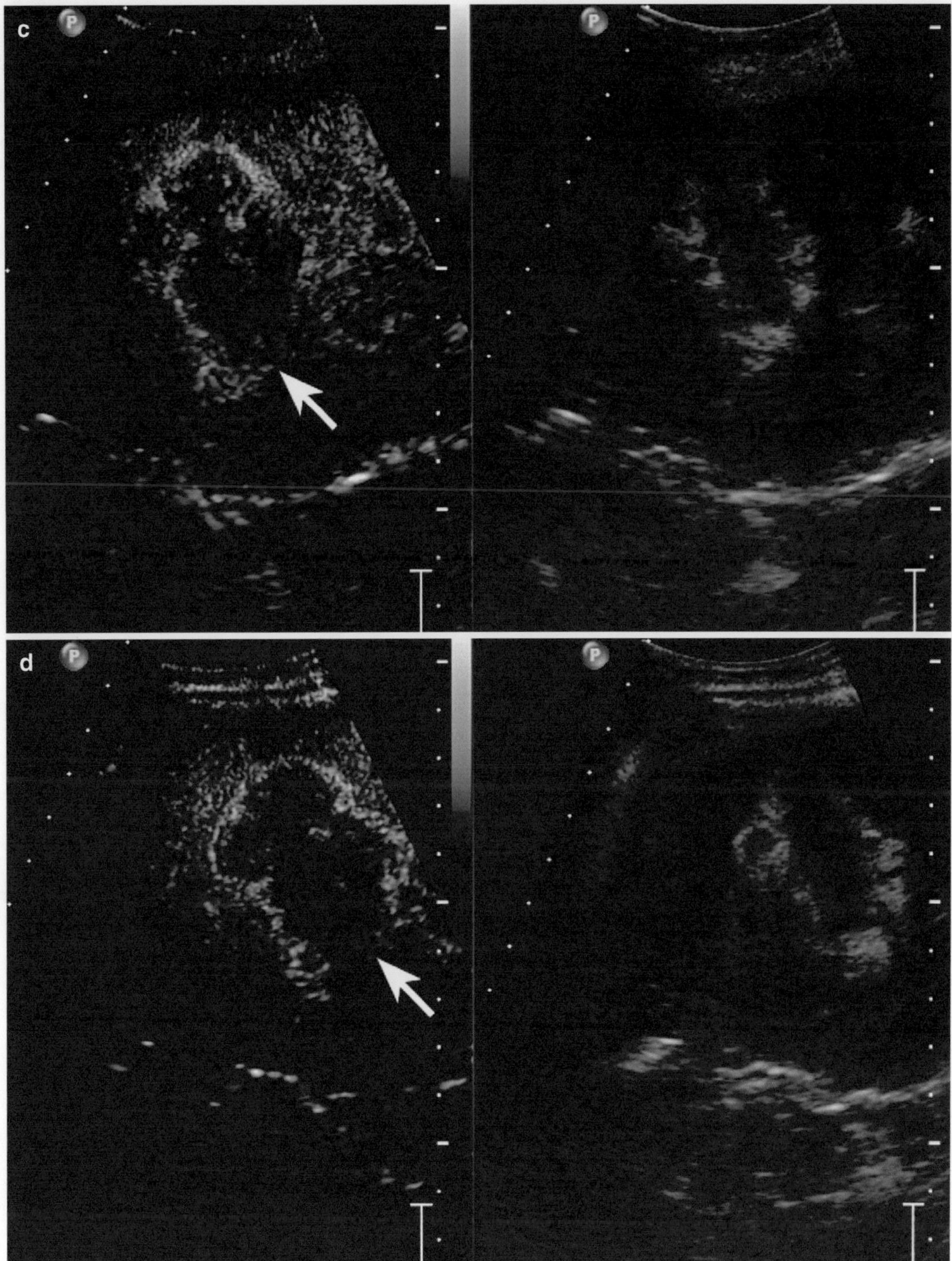

Fig. 3.12 (continued)

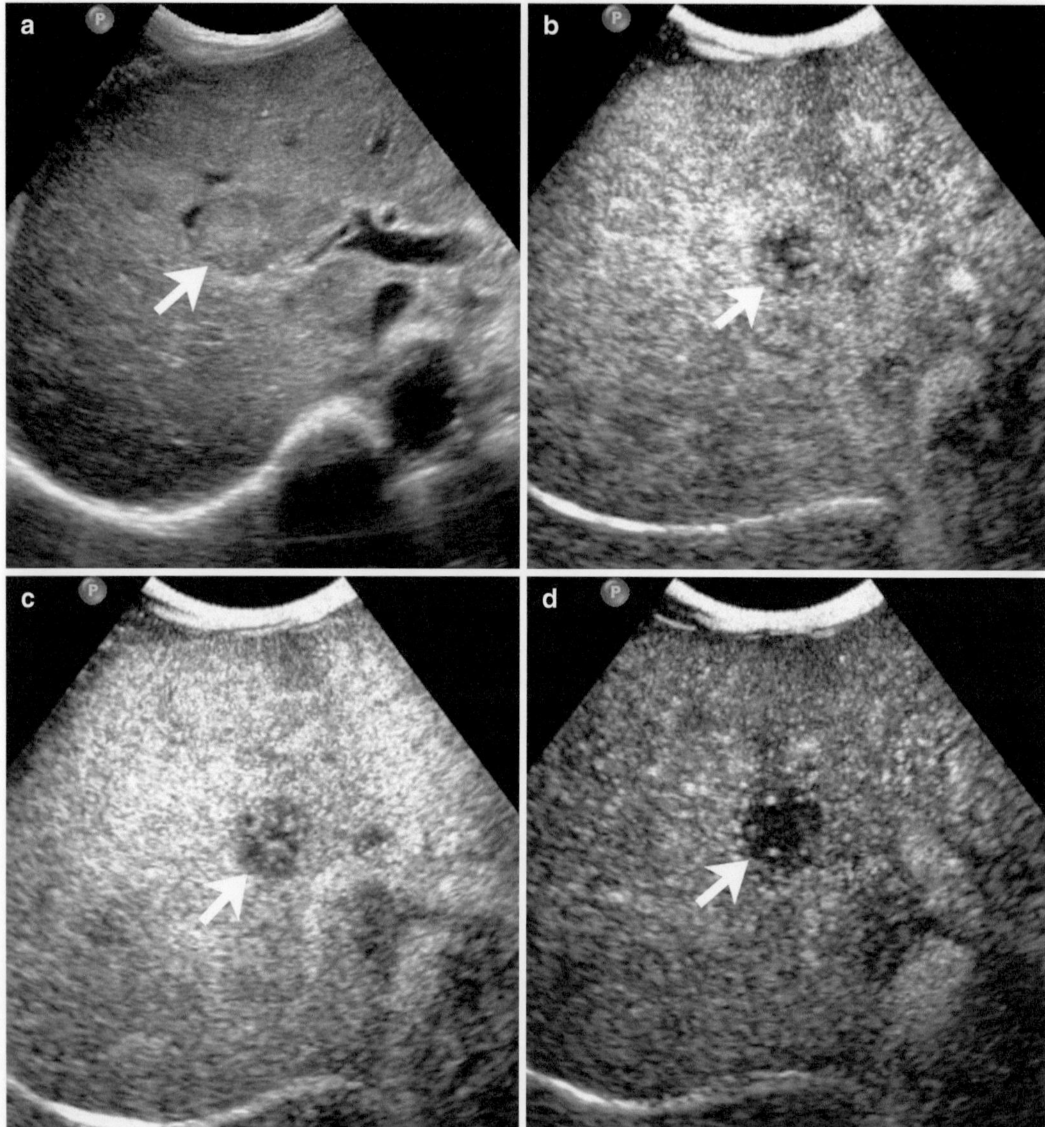

Fig. 3.13 Metastasis with "dotted" appearance in a 76-year-old woman. (**a**) Oblique ascending right subcostal baseline image reveals an inhomogeneous slightly hypoechoic lesion sized 2 cm in the V hepatic segment (*arrow*). (**b**) In the arterial phase, several hypervascular spots are appreciable within the lesion (*arrow*). (**c**, **d**) In portal-venous and late phase images, the lesion shows a progressive washout and appears mainly hypoechoic with respect to the surrounding hepatic parenchyma (*arrows*)

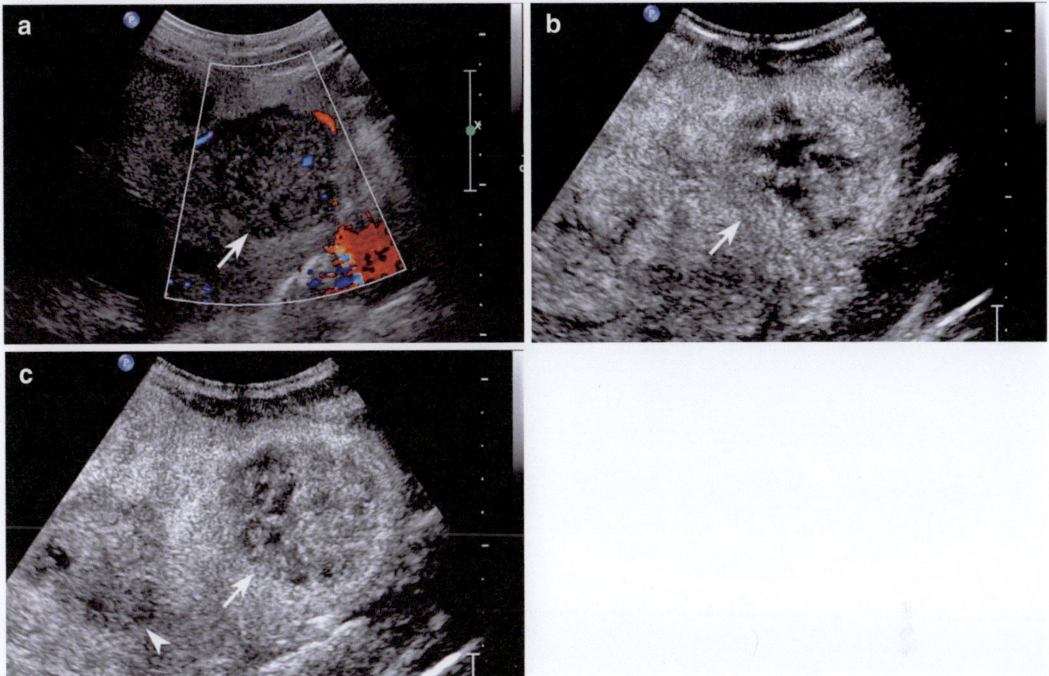

Fig. 3.14 Metastases from Gastrointestinal stromal tumors (GIST) in a 42-year-old man. (**a**) Baseline US image shows a markedly inhomogeneous hypoechoic lesion sized 4.5 cm in the left lobe with vascular signal within the mass at color-Doppler study (*arrow*). (**b**) At CEUS, the lesion appears highly and inhomogeneously hypervascular in the arterial phase with rapid washout in the portal-venous (**c**) phase (*arrows*). Another similar lesion is evident in this scan (*arrowhead*)

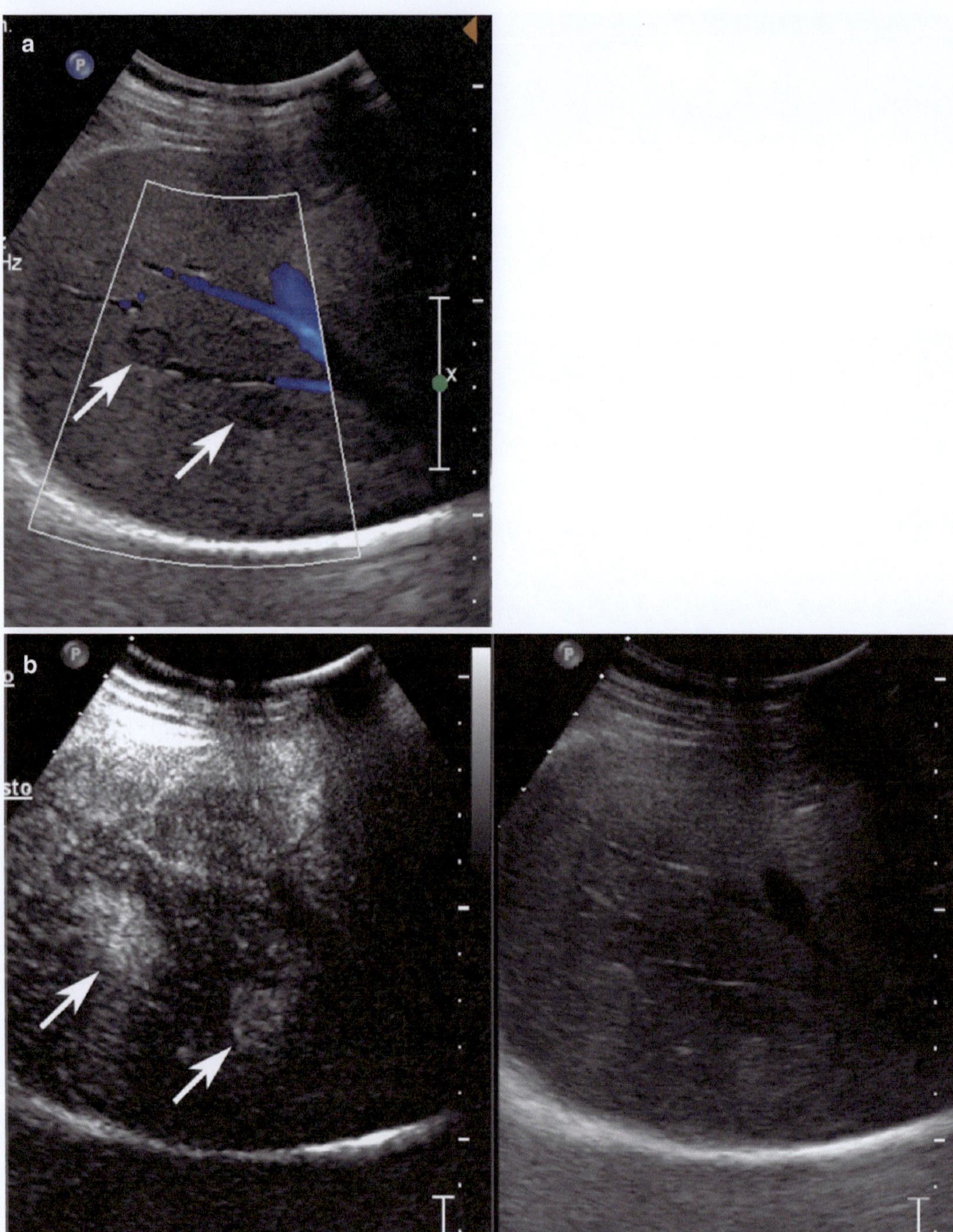

Fig. 3.15 Liver metastases from melanoma in a 35-year-old woman. (**a**) Oblique ascending right subcostal baseline image reveals two well-defined 1 cm-sized lesions in the VII hepatic segment, isoechoic in the central portion with tiny peripheral hypoechoic rim not showing vascular signal at color-Doppler evaluation (*arrows*). (**b**) In the arterial phase, the lesions show a clear-cut contrast uptake (*arrows*) with evident washout in the portal-venous (**c**) and late (**d**) phases (*arrows*)

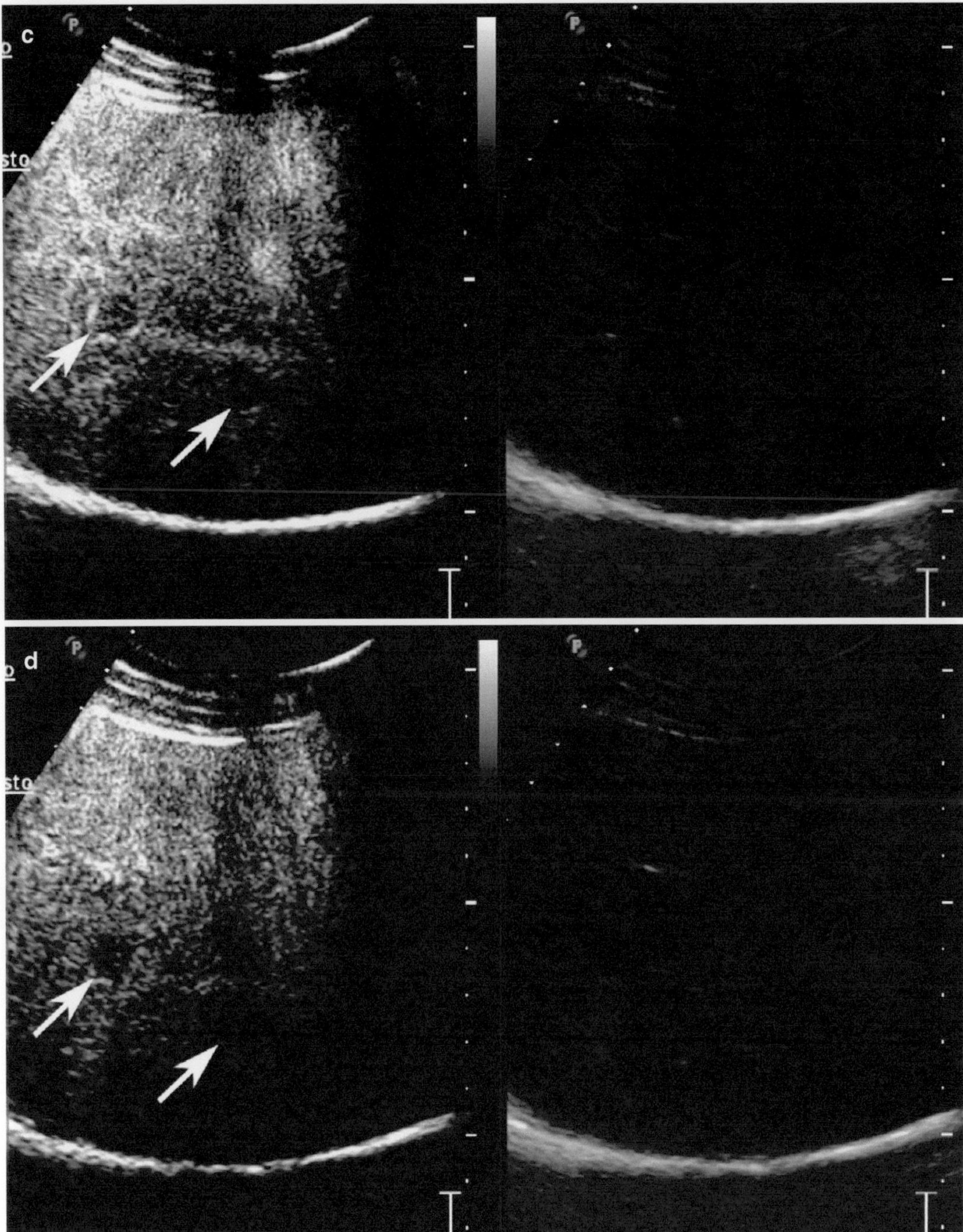

Fig. 3.15 (continued)

3.3.2   Hypovascular Metastases

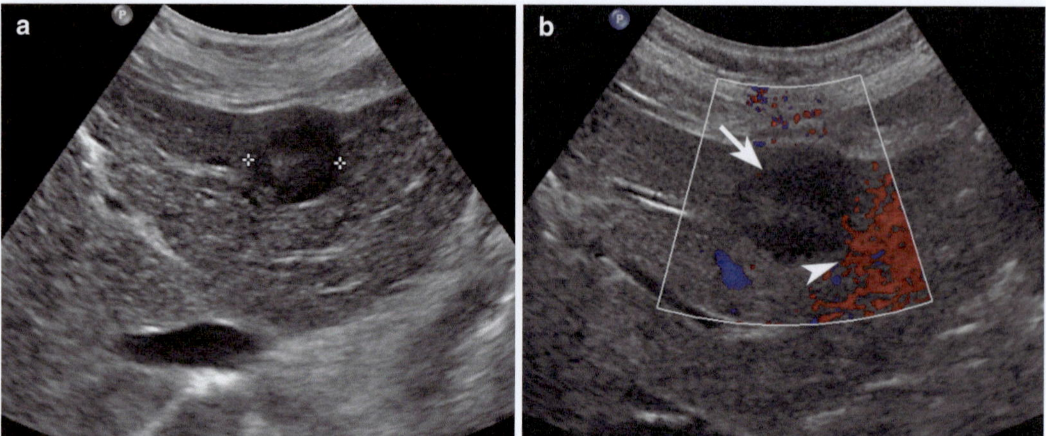

Fig. 3.16 MTS in a 55-year-old woman with pancreatic adenocarcinoma. (**a**) Subcostal right baseline image reveals an hypoechoic lesion sized 4.2 cm in the III–IV hepatic segment (*calipers*). (**b**) The mass does not show any vascular signal at color-Doppler evaluation (*arrow*). Conspicuous cardiac pulsatility artifacts are evident (*arrowhead*). At CEUS, the lesion shows mainly peripheral enhancement around a marked hypoechoic area in the arterial phase (*arrow*) (**c**) and maintains inhomogeneous aspect in the extended portal venous phase (**d**) (*arrow*)

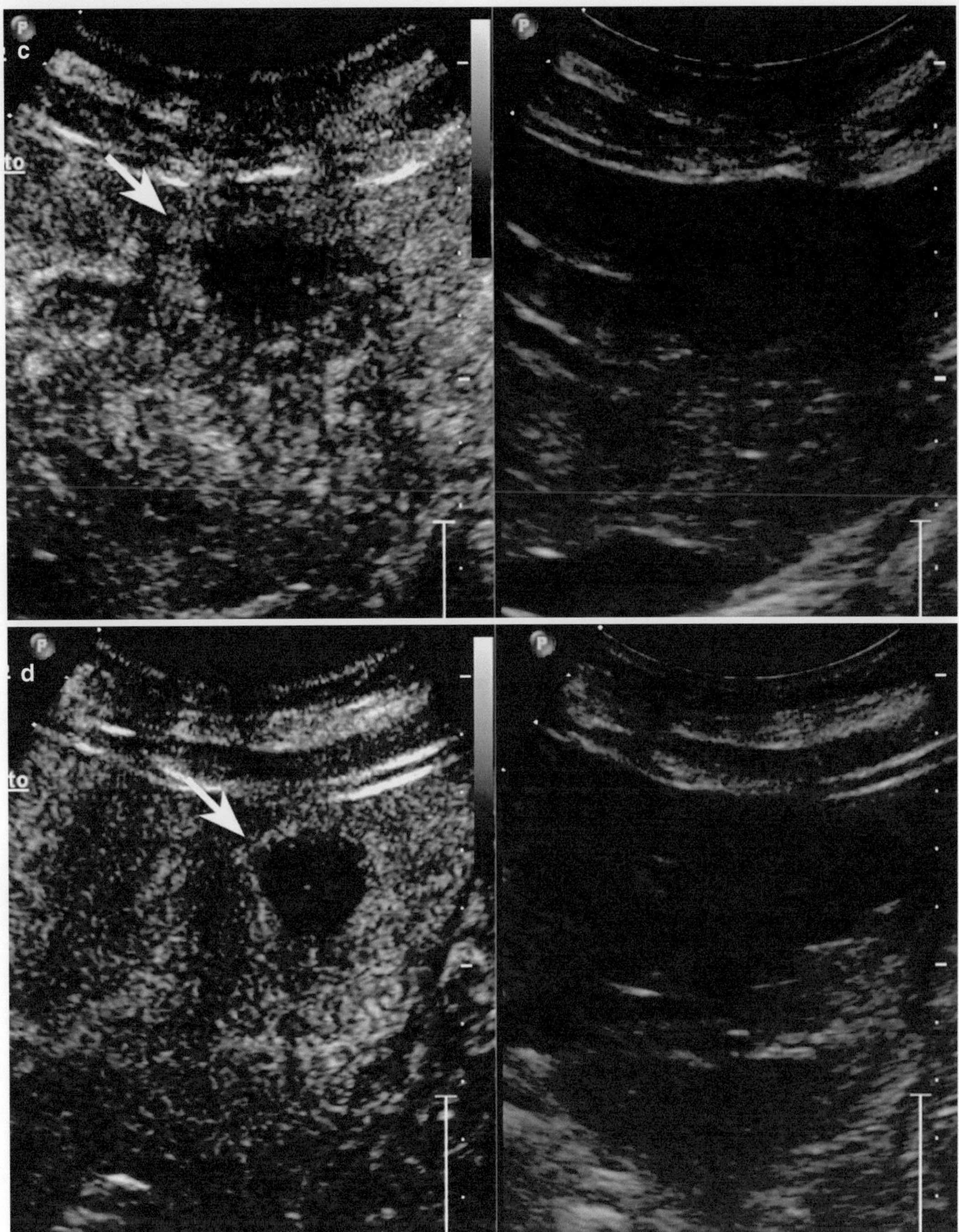

Fig. 3.16 (continued)

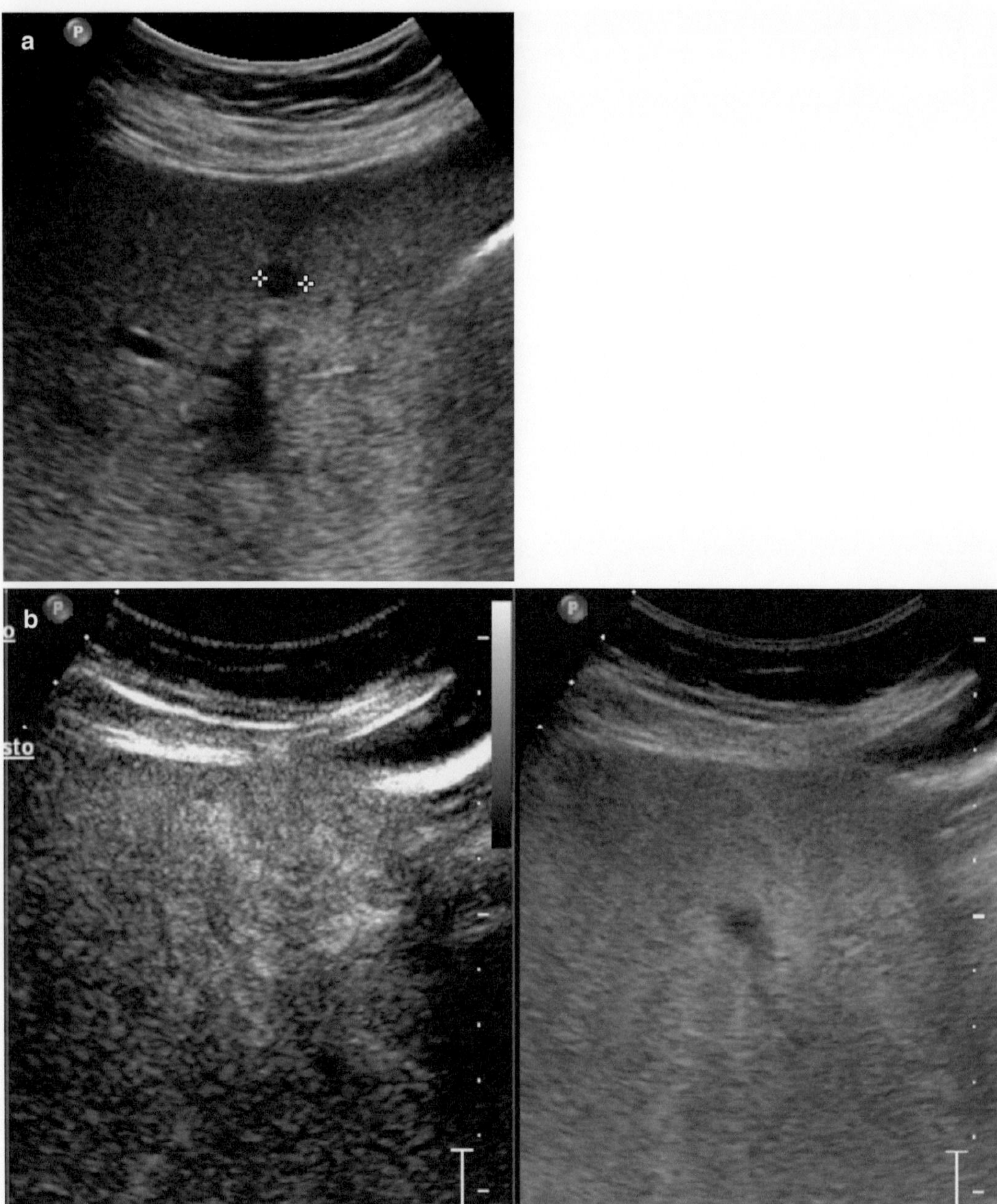

Fig. 3.17 Liver metastasis from breast cancer. (**a**) Oblique ascending right subcostal baseline image in a 57-year-old woman shows a 9 mm-sized homogeneous hypoechoic lesion in fatty liver located in the IV hepatic segment (*arrow*). (**b**) The lesion presents isoechoic with respect to the surrounding liver parenchyma in the arterial phase showing a clear-cut washout in the portal-venous (**c**) and late phases (**d**) (*arrows*)

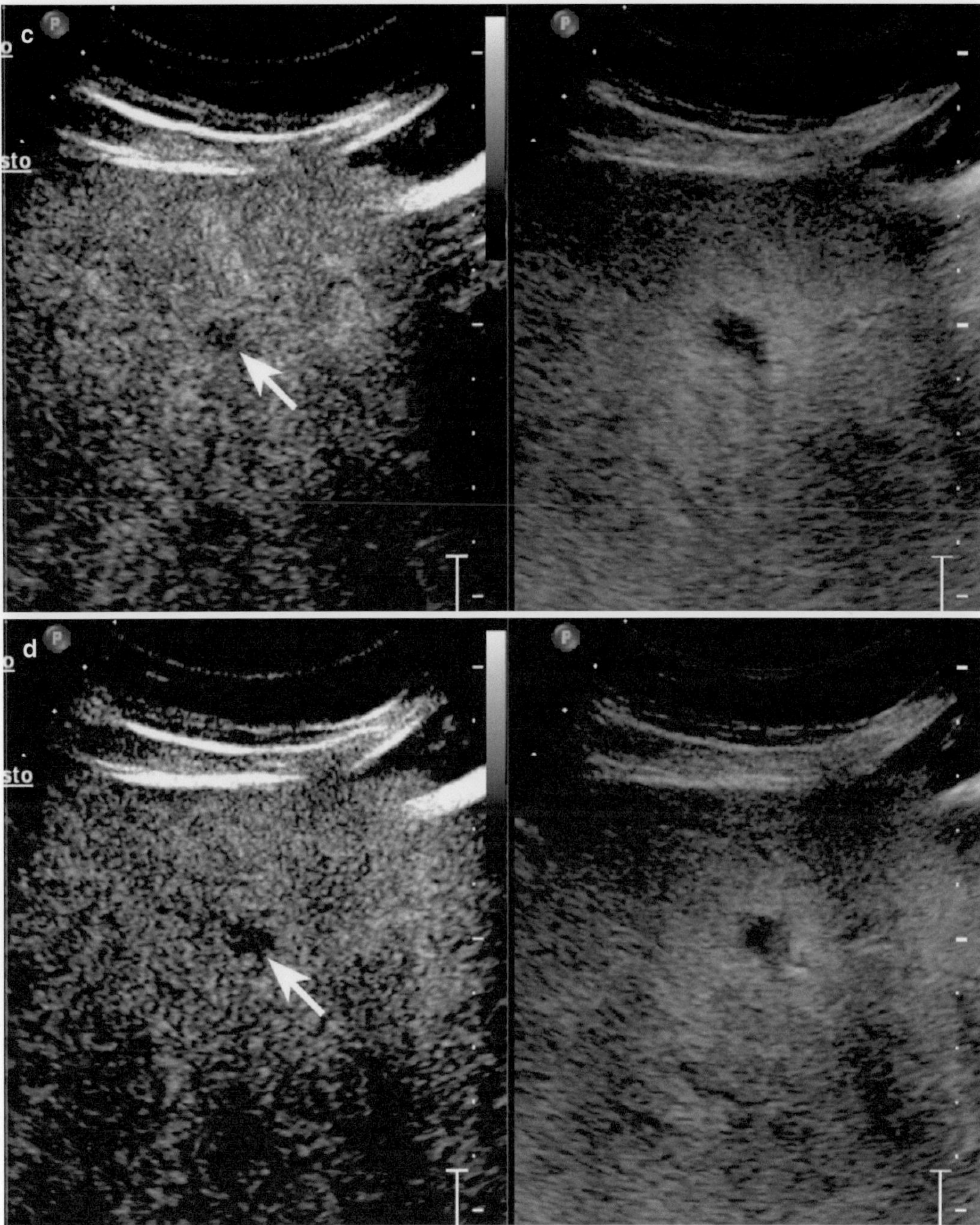

Fig. 3.17 (continued)

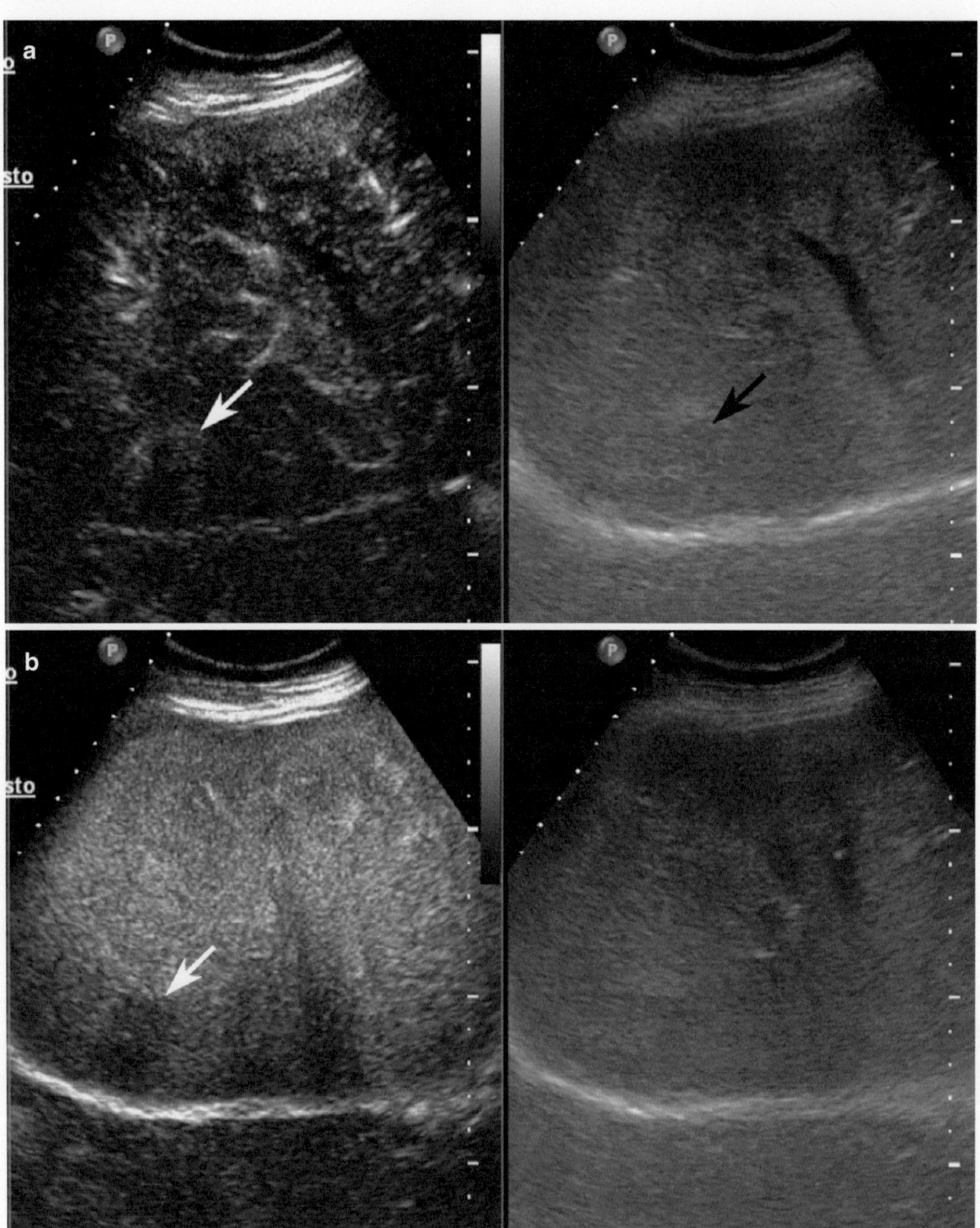

Fig. 3.18 Liver metastasis from rectal cancer in a 72-year-old man. (**a**) Unenhanced US image reveals a slightly hypoechoic lesion sized 3.5 cm in the VII hepatic segment (*black arrow*; *right side*). The mass presents an inhomogeneous peripheral rim enhancement in the arterial phase (*white arrow*; *left side*) with a clear-cut washout in the portal-venous (**b**) and late phases (**c**) (*arrows*)

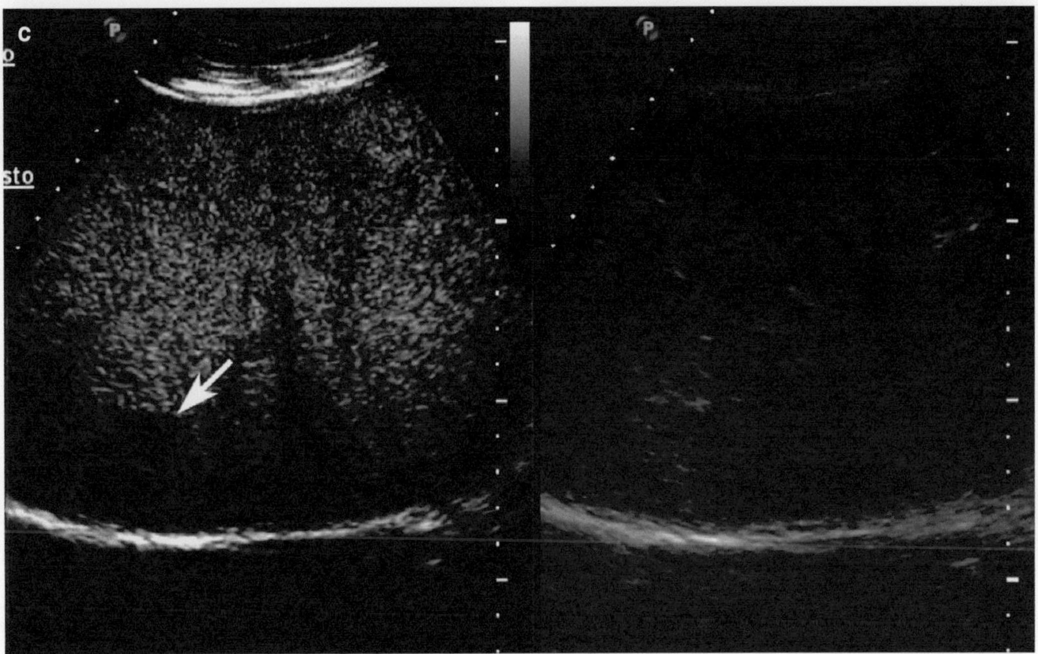

Fig. 3.18 (continued)

References

Intrahepatic Cholangiocarcinoma

1. Ros PR, Menu Y, Vilgrain V (2001) Liver neoplasms and tumor-like conditions. Eur Radiol 11:S145–S165
2. Loria F, Loria G, Basile S, Crea G, Frosina L, Di Carlo I (2014) Contrast-enhanced ultrasound appearances of enhancement patterns of intrahepatic cholangiocarcinoma: correlation with pathological findings. Updates Surg 66:135–143
3. Bauditz J, Schade T, Wermke W (2007) Sonographic diagnosis of hilar cholangiocarcinomas by the use of cont rast agents. Ultraschall Med 28:161–167

FLLs in Cirrhotic Patients

4. Bhosale P, Szklaruk J, Silverman PM (2006) Current staging of hepatocellular carcinoma: imaging implications. Cancer Imaging 6:83–94
5. Hussain SM, Zondervan PE, Ijzermans JN, Schalm SW, de Man RA, Krestin GP (2002) Benign versus malignant hepatic nodules: MR imaging findings with pathologic correlation. Radiographics 22:1023–1036
6. Nakashima Y, Nakashima O, Hsia CC, Kojiro M, Tabor E (1999) Vascularization of small hepatocellular carcinomas: correlation with differentiation. Liver 19:12–18
7. Jang HJ, Kim TK, Burns PN, Wilson SR (2007) Enhancement patterns of hepatocellular carcinoma at contrast-enhanced US: comparison with histologic differentiation. Radiology 244:898–906
8. Kudo M (2006) Early detection and characterization of hepatocellular carcinoma: value of imaging multistep human hepatocarcinogenesis. Intervirology 49:64–69
9. Kim TK, Jang HJ (2014) Contrast-enhanced ultrasound in the diagnosis of nodules in liver cirrhosis. World J Gastroenterol 20:3590–3596
10. Wilson SR, Kim TK, Jang HJ, Burns PN (2007) Enhancement patterns of focal liver masses: discordance between contrast-enhanced sonography and contrast-enhanced CT and MRI. AJR Am J Roentgenol 189:W7–W12
11. Wilson SR, Burns PN (2006) An algorithm for the diagnosis of focal liver masses using microbubble contrast-enhanced pulse-inversion sonography. AJR Am J Roentgenol 186:1401–1412

Metastases

12. Garden OJ, Rees M, Poston GJ, Mirza D, Saunders M, Ledermann J, Primrose JN, Parks RW (2006) Guidelines for resection of colorectal cancer liver metastases. Gut 55(Suppl 3):iii1–iii8
13. Rappeport ED, Loft A, Berthelsen AK, von der Recke P, Larsen PN, Mogensen AM, Wettergren A, Rasmussen A, Hillingsoe J, Kirkegaard P, Thomsen C (2007) Contrast-enhanced FDG-PET/CT vs. SPIO-enhanced MRI vs. FDG-PET vs. CT in patients with liver metastases from colorectal cancer: a prospective study with intraoperative confirmation. Acta Radiol 48:369–378
14. Cantisani V, Grazhdani H, Fioravanti C, Rosignuolo M, Calliada F, Messineo D et al (2014) Liver metastases: contrast-enhanced ultrasound compared with computed tomography and magnetic resonance. World J Gastroenterol 20(29):9998–10007
15. Bang N, Bolvig L, Christiansen T, Laurberg S (2007) The value of contrast enhanced ultrasonography in detection of liver metastases from colorectal cancer: a prospective double-blinded study. Eur J Radiol 62:302–327
16. Janica JR, Lebkowska U, Ustymowicz A, Augustynowicz A, Kamocki Z, Werel D (2007) Contrast-enhanced ultrasonography in diagnosing liver metastases. Med Sci Monit 13(Suppl 1):111–115
17. Konopke R, Bunk A, Kersting S (2007) The role of contrast-enhanced ultrasound for focal liver lesion detection: an overview. Ultrasound Med Biol 33:1515–1526
18. Murphy-Lavallee J, Jang HJ, Kim TK, Burns PN, Wilson SR (2007) Are metastases really hypovascular in the arterial phase? The perspective based on contrast-enhanced ultrasonography. J Ultrasound Med 26:1545–1556

Fatty Liver, Pseudolesions

4

Diffuse fatty infiltration is a common imaging finding due to the abnormal accumulation of lipids within hepatocytes. Baseline US is typically the first imaging modality for the evaluation of hepatic steatosis, but causing a conspicuous increase in liver echogenicity and a marked ultrasound beam attenuation, it really hampers FLL detection and characterization. Moreover, geographic fatty changes of the liver can occur when the fat accumulation ability of hepatocytes or fat deposition becomes heterogeneous throughout the liver and are classified into four subtypes: (a) focal fatty change, (b) multifocal steatosis, (c) lobar or segmental steatosis, and (d) focal fatty sparing in fatty liver [1].

In particular, focal fatty change and focal fatty sparing can show a round, mass-like appearance on imaging, making difficult a correct differential diagnosis with malignant lesions in oncological patients. At this regard, CEUS has been reported to improve the characterization of focal hepatic lesions in patients with fatty liver and in diagnosing both focal fatty infiltration and sparing [2]. But there are different and controversial data in literature about the usefulness of CEUS in the screening and follow-up of oncological patients [3–9]. Anyway, WFUMB-EFSUMB guidelines recommend CEUS in the surveillance of oncological patients (if CEUS has been useful previously), for the evaluation of liver metastases in colorectal cancer after chemotherapy instead of unenhanced US, or for lesion(s) or suspected lesion(s) detected with US in patients with a known history of a malignancy as an alternative to CT or MRI [10–12].

© Springer International Publishing Switzerland 2015
T.V. Bartolotta et al., *Atlas of Contrast-enhanced Sonography of Focal Liver Lesions*,
DOI 10.1007/978-3-319-17539-3_4

4.1   Diffuse Fatty Liver

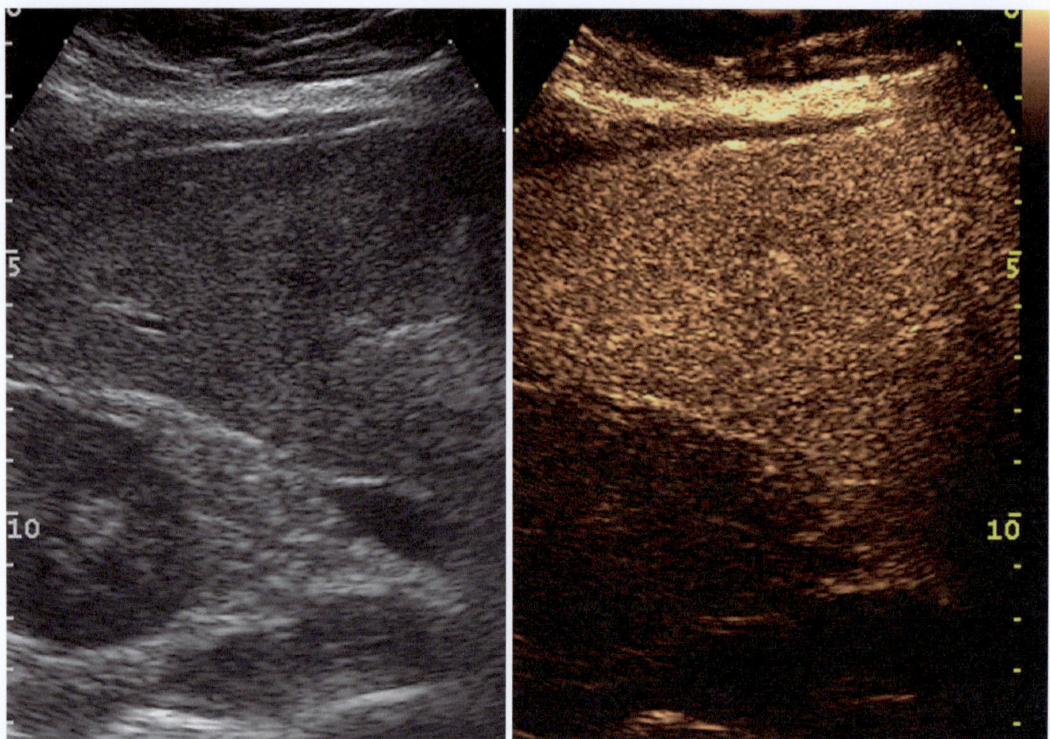

Fig. 4.1 Diffuse fatty change in a 65-year-old man. At unenhanced US (*left image*), diffuse fatty change is appreciable. At CEUS (*right image*), homogeneous contrast enhancement is evident in the extended portal-venous phase

4.2 **Geographic Fatty Change**

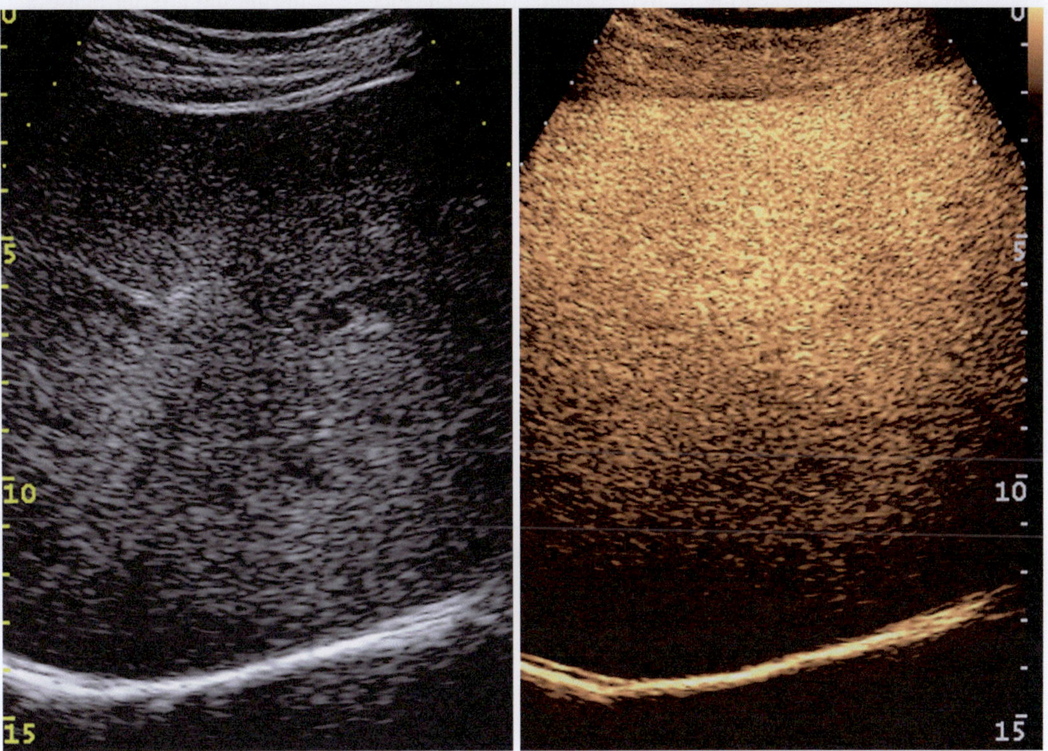

Fig. 4.2 Geographic fatty change in a 49-year-old woman. At unenhanced US (*left image*), diffuse inhomogeneous fatty infiltration is evident. At CEUS (*right image*), homogenous contrast enhancement is evident in the extended portal-venous phase

4.3   Focal Fatty Change

Focal fatty changes—presenting as hyperechoic areas in otherwise normal liver—and focal sparing areas—occurring as hypoechoic areas in a diffuse fatty "bright liver"—usually show no differences in contrast uptake in comparison with adjacent liver parenchyma. Consequently, at CEUS, these "pseudolesions" do not show contrast enhancement during the arterial phase and become isoechoic in comparison with the surrounding liver parenchyma in the extended portal-venous phase [13].

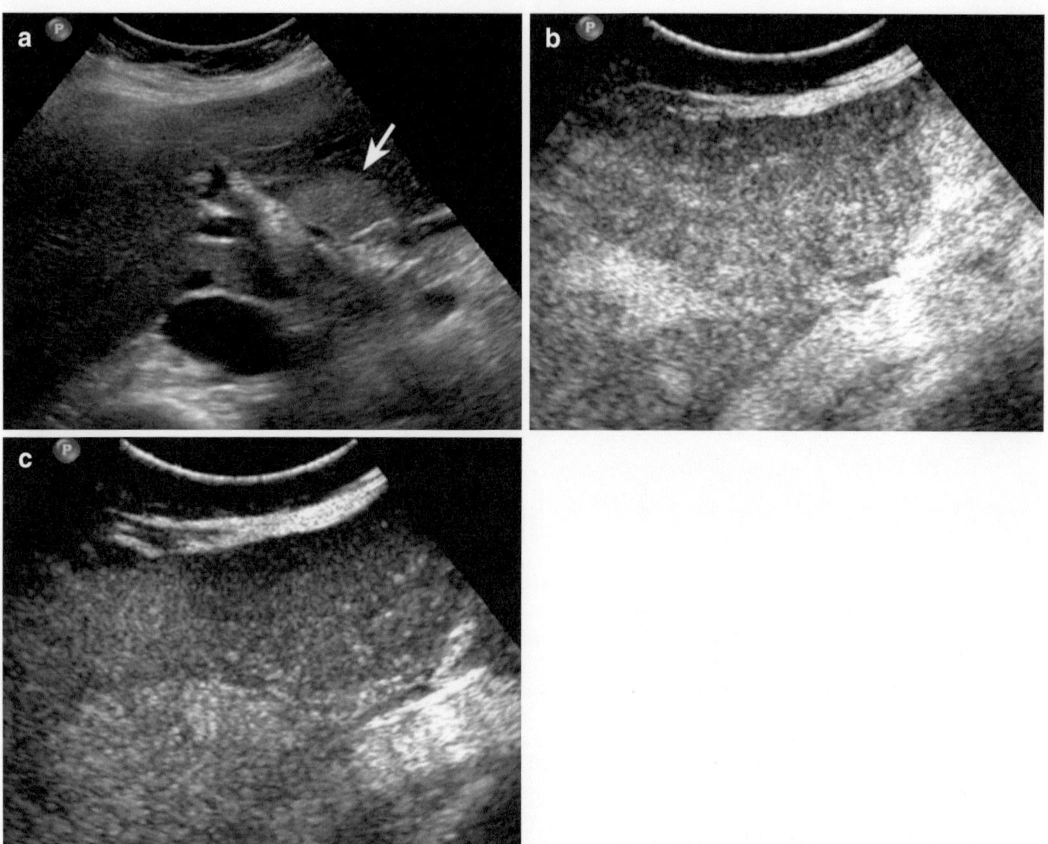

Fig. 4.3 Focal fatty area in a 58-year-old man. (**a**) At baseline US, an hyperechoic area sized 3.5 cm is detected in segment IV (*arrow*). (**b**, **c**) At CEUS, the area is evident neither in the arterial phase (**b**) nor in the late phase (**c**)

4.4 Focal Sparing

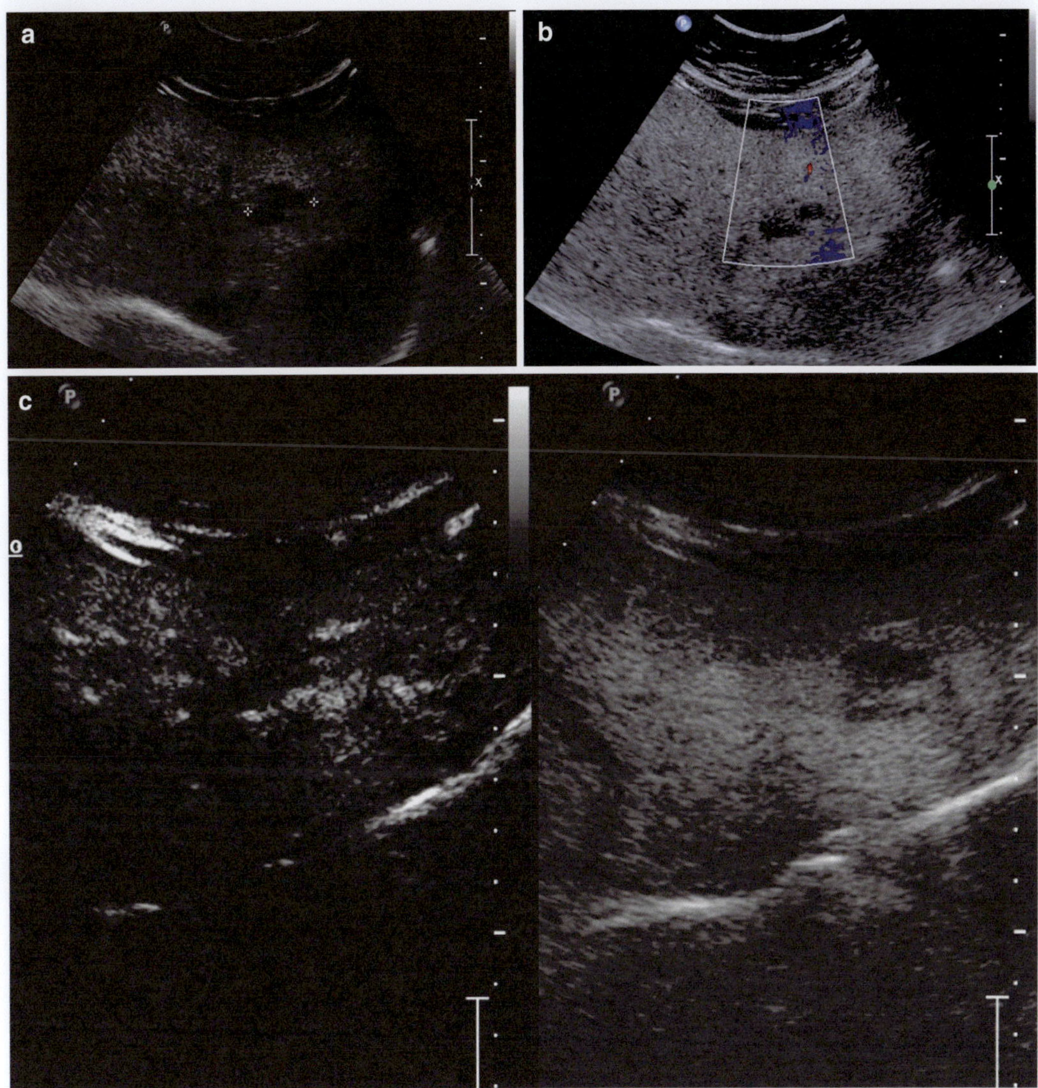

Fig. 4.4 Focal fatty sparing in a 48-year-old asymptomatic woman. (**a**) Transverse baseline US image reveals a 2.4 cm hypoechoic area in the IV hepatic segment (calipers) without vascular signal at color-Doppler evaluation (**b**). At CEUS, the pseudolesion shows the same contrast enhancement of the adjacent liver parenchyma during the arterial (**c**), portal-venous (**d**), and late (**e**) phases

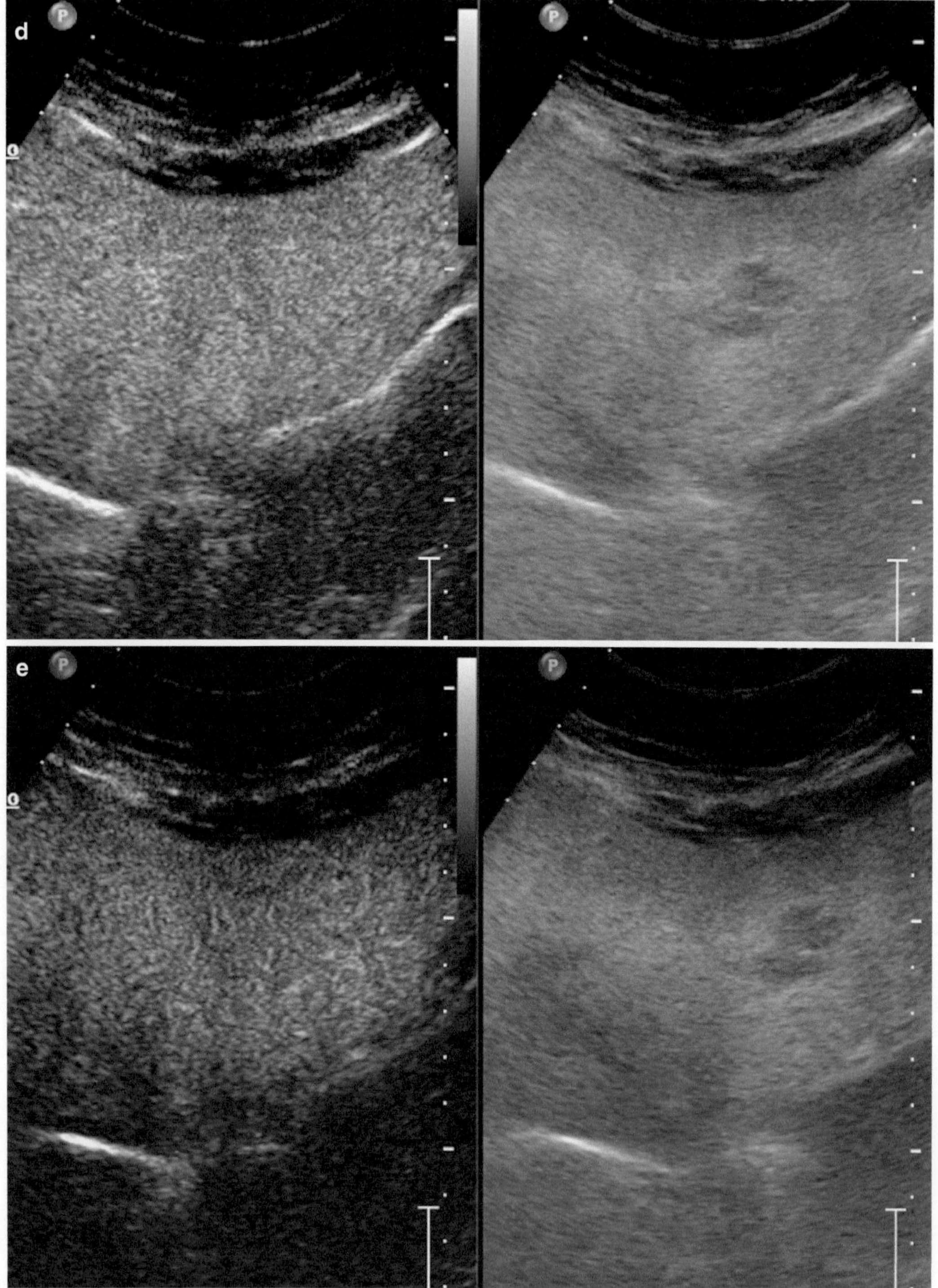

Fig. 4.4 (continued)

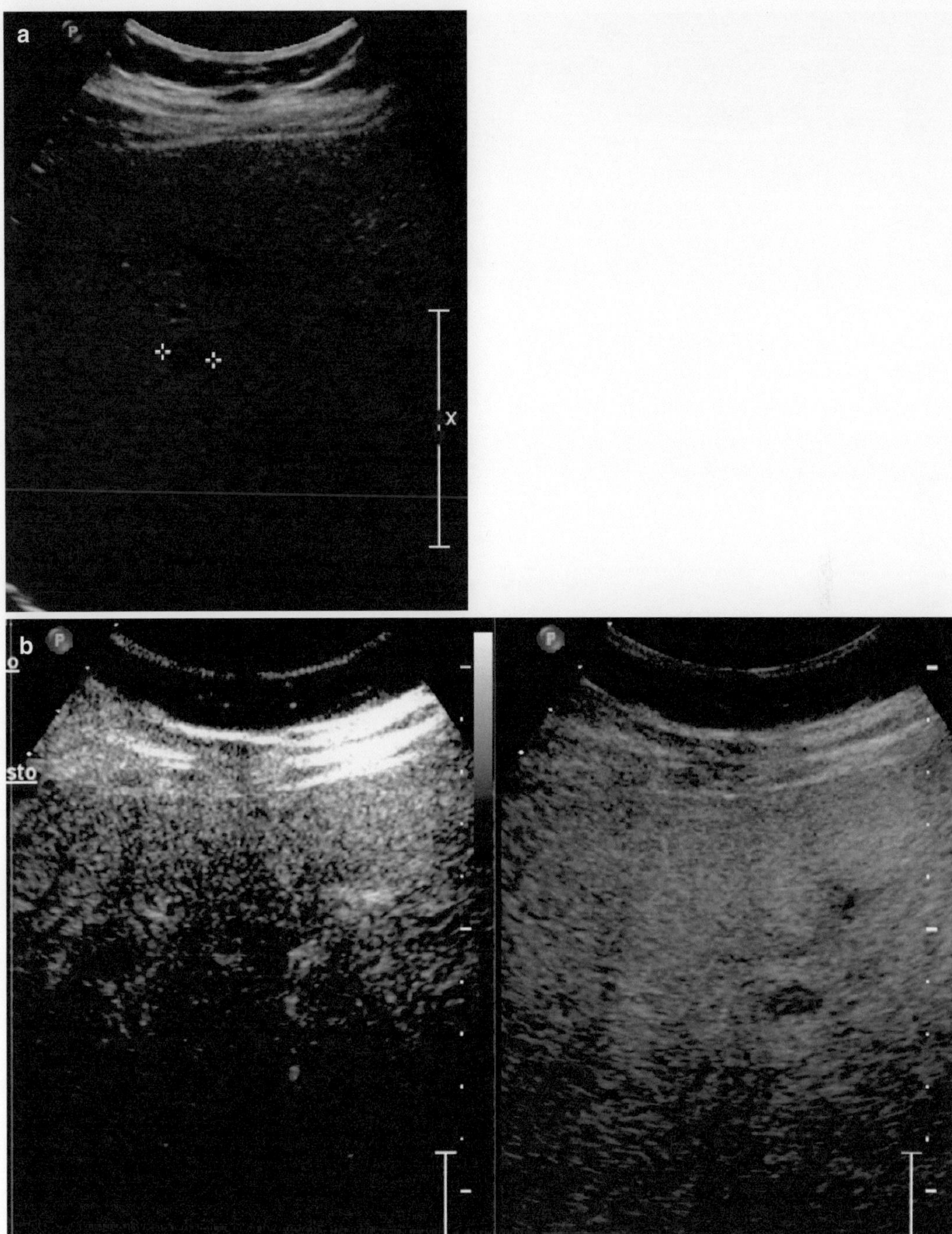

Fig. 4.5 Nodular focal fatty sparing in a 48-year-old woman with colon cancer. (**a**) Oblique ascending baseline US image reveals a 1.2 cm hypoechoic nodular area in the VII hepatic segment in fatty liver (calipers). (**b–d**) At CEUS, the pseudolesion is not evident throughout the vascular study

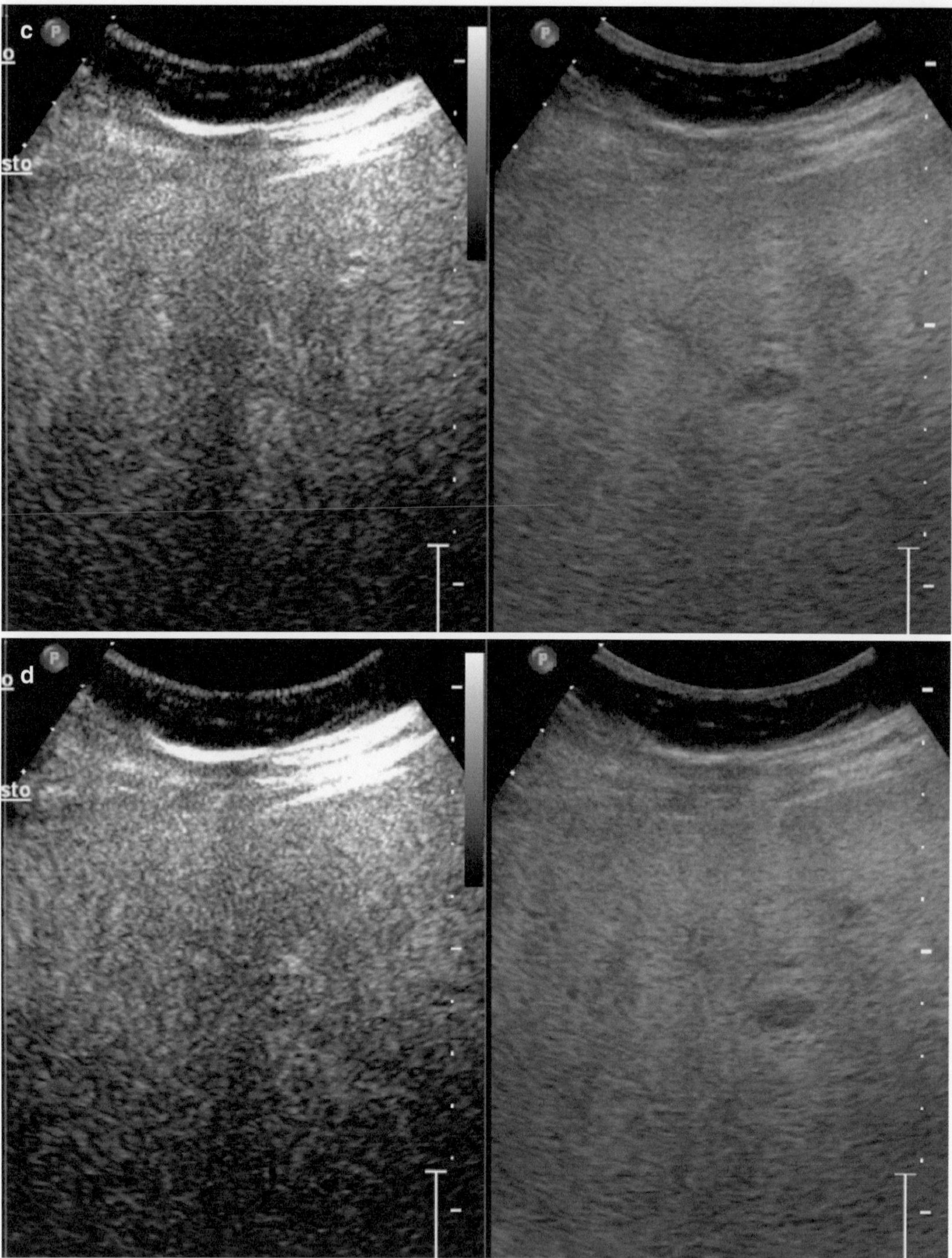

Fig. 4.5 (continued)

4.5 Focal Liver Lesions in Fatty Liver

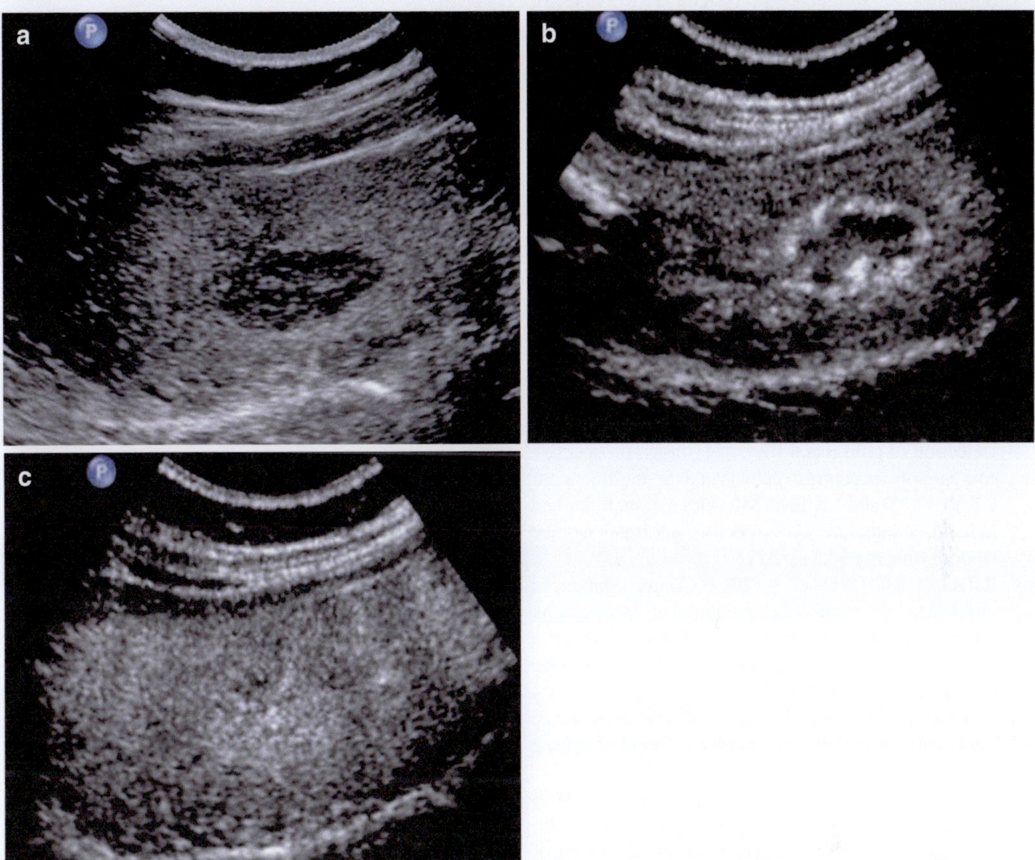

Fig. 4.6 Liver hemangioma in fatty liver in 55-year-old man. (**a**) Right subcostal oblique ascending scan shows an inhomogeneous hypoechoic 3.5 cm-sized lesion with well-defined margins in segment VIII, indeterminate at baseline US. (**b**) In the arterial phase, the lesion shows peripheral globular enhancement with progressive centripetal fill-in, complete in the extended portal-venous phase (**c**)

References

1. Shiozawa K, Watanabe M, Ikehara T, Kogame M, Shinohara M, Shinohara M et al (2014) Evaluation of hemodynamics in focal steatosis and focal spared lesion of the liver using contrast-enhanced ultrasonography with sonazoid. Radiol Res Pract: 604594. doi:10.1155/2014/604594
2. Janica J, Ustymowicz A, Lukasiewicz A et al (2013) Comparison of contrast-enhanced ultrasonography with grey-scale ultrasonography and contrast-enhanced computed tomography in diagnosing focal fatty liver infiltrations and focal fatty sparing. Adv Med Sci 58:408–418
3. Konopke R, Bunk A, Kersting S (2008) Contrast-enhanced ultrasonography in patients with colorectal liver metastases after chemotherapy. Ultraschall Med 29(Suppl 4):S203–S209
4. Mainenti PP, Mancini M, Mainolfi C et al (2010) Detection of colo-rectal liver metastases: prospective comparison of contrast enhanced US, multidetector CT, PET/CT, and 1.5 Tesla MR with extracellular and reticulo-endothelial cell specific contrast agents. Abdom Imaging 35:511–521
5. Rafaelsen SR, Jakobsen A (2011) Contrast-enhanced ultrasound vs multidetector-computed tomography for detecting liver metastases in colorectal cancer: a prospective, blinded, patient-by-patient analysis. Colorectal Dis 13:420–425
6. Nicolau C, Ripollés T (2012) Contrast-enhanced ultrasound in abdominal imaging. Abdom Imaging 37:1–19
7. Larsen LP, Rosenkilde M, Christensen H et al (2009) Can contrast-enhanced ultrasonography replace multidetector-computed tomography in the detection of liver metastases from colorectal cancer? Eur J Radiol 69:308–313
8. Muhi A, Ichikawa T, Motosugi U et al (2011) Diagnosis of colorectal hepatic metastases: comparison of contrast-enhanced CT, contrast-enhanced US, superparamagnetic iron oxide-enhanced MRI, and gadoxetic acid-enhanced MRI. J Magn Reson Imaging 34:326–335
9. Cabassa P, Bipat S, Longaretti L et al (2010) Liver metastases: sulphur hexafluoride-enhanced ultrasonography for lesion detection: a systematic review. Ultrasound Med Biol 36:1561–1567
10. Claudon M, Dietrich CF, Choi BI, Cosgrove DO, Kudo M, Nolsøe CP et al (2013) Guidelines and good clinical practice recommendations for contrast enhanced ultrasound (CEUS) in the liver – update 2012. A WFUMB-EFSUMB initiative in cooperation with representatives of AFSUMB, AIUM, ASUM, FLAUS and ICUS. Ultraschall Med 34:11–29
11. Bartolotta TV, Taibbi A, Galia M, Runza G, Matranga D, Midiri M, Lagalla R (2007) Characterization of hypoechoic focal hepatic lesions in patients with fatty liver: diagnostic performance and confidence of contrast-enhanced ultrasound. Eur Radiol 17(3):650–661
12. Bartolotta TV, Midiri M, Scialpi M, Sciarrino E, Galia M, Lagalla R (2004) Focal nodular hyperplasia in normal and fatty liver: a qualitative and quantitative evaluation with contrast-enhanced ultrasound. Eur Radiol 14(4):583–591

Focal Fatty Change

13. Bartolotta TV, Taibbi A, Midiri M, Lagalla R (2009) Focal liver lesions:contrast-enhanced ultrasound. Abdom Imaging 34(2):193–209

5.1   Angiomyolipoma

The angiomyolipoma (AML) is a mixed mesenchymal tumor that rarely arises in the liver, being more frequent in the kidney. It presents as single or multiple lesions. It is constituted from smooth muscle cells, adipocytes, and blood vessels in variable percentages influencing imaging appearance. AML is benign and rarely evolves into a malignant form with invasion of adjacent vessels and metastases in the omental zone [1]. The preoperative diagnosis is not easy because of the not-infrequent overlapping findings with other benign or malignant lesions with fatty content [2]. The size can vary from few millimeters up to 30 cm, so AML can be an incidental finding in asymptomatic patients or, in large lesions, presents with abdominal pain due to compression of adjacent structures or rupture with bleeding [3].

At US, the lesion appears with well-defined margins, not encapsulated, inhomogeneous, mainly hyperechoic. At color-Doppler, vascularity is poorly represented, and some intralesional and peripheral arterial vascular signals can be observed [2, 4, 5].

After administration of ultrasound contrast agent AML shows, in the arterial phase, early and marked enhancement except for fatty areas. The contrast enhancement pattern is variable in the extended portal venous phase. Some authors described the persistence of contrast medium uptake, but "washout" was reported too, making difficult a correct differentiation with other hypervascular lesions containing fat as HCC or liver liposarcoma [6]. So CEUS examination can be useful in highlighting the hypervascularity in the arterial phase, but biopsy or surgical removal of the mass are often mandatory in order to obtain the final diagnosis.

© Springer International Publishing Switzerland 2015
T.V. Bartolotta et al., *Atlas of Contrast-enhanced Sonography of Focal Liver Lesions*,
DOI 10.1007/978-3-319-17539-3_5

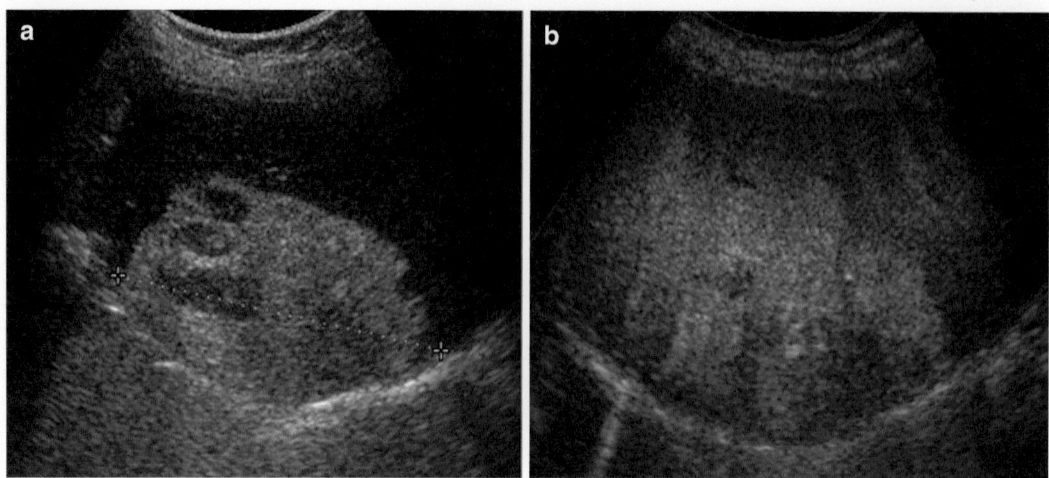

Fig. 5.1 Hepatic angiomyolipoma. (**a**) Right subcostal ascending US scan shows in segment VII a wide markedly hyperechoic lesion with regular margins (calipers) and some small hyperechoic area in the context. (**b**) After contrast medium injection, the lesion appears inhomogeneously hypervascular

5.2 Solitary Necrotic Nodule

The solitary necrotic nodule (SNN) is a rare benign tumor of uncertain origin often incidentally discovered. According to some authors, it represents a natural evolution of traumatic injury, infection by parasites, or a sclerosing hemangioma and can present as single or multiple lesions and is often misinterpreted as metastasis [7–9]. At microscopic examination, it can show different aspects: (1) an area of central coagulation necrosis often partially calcified, surrounded by a fibrous capsule in which inflammatory cells can also be evident; (2) coagulation necrosis mixed with liquefactive necrosis; and (3) multinodular fusion [10].

At US, SNN appears mainly hypoechoic and can show a "target" aspect with a central hyperechoic area and calcifications. According to literature, US aspect depends on the homogeneity of necrosis and the degree of dehydration of the lesion. Usually, it has a bilobed or polilobulated form, unusual for metastases, and grows in proximity to vascular structures. At color-Doppler, it shows no signal [9, 11]. After administration of USCA, SNN does not show substantial changes throughout the vascular phases, and as reported in literature, it shows mild or moderate enhancement at CT and MR [10, 12, 13].

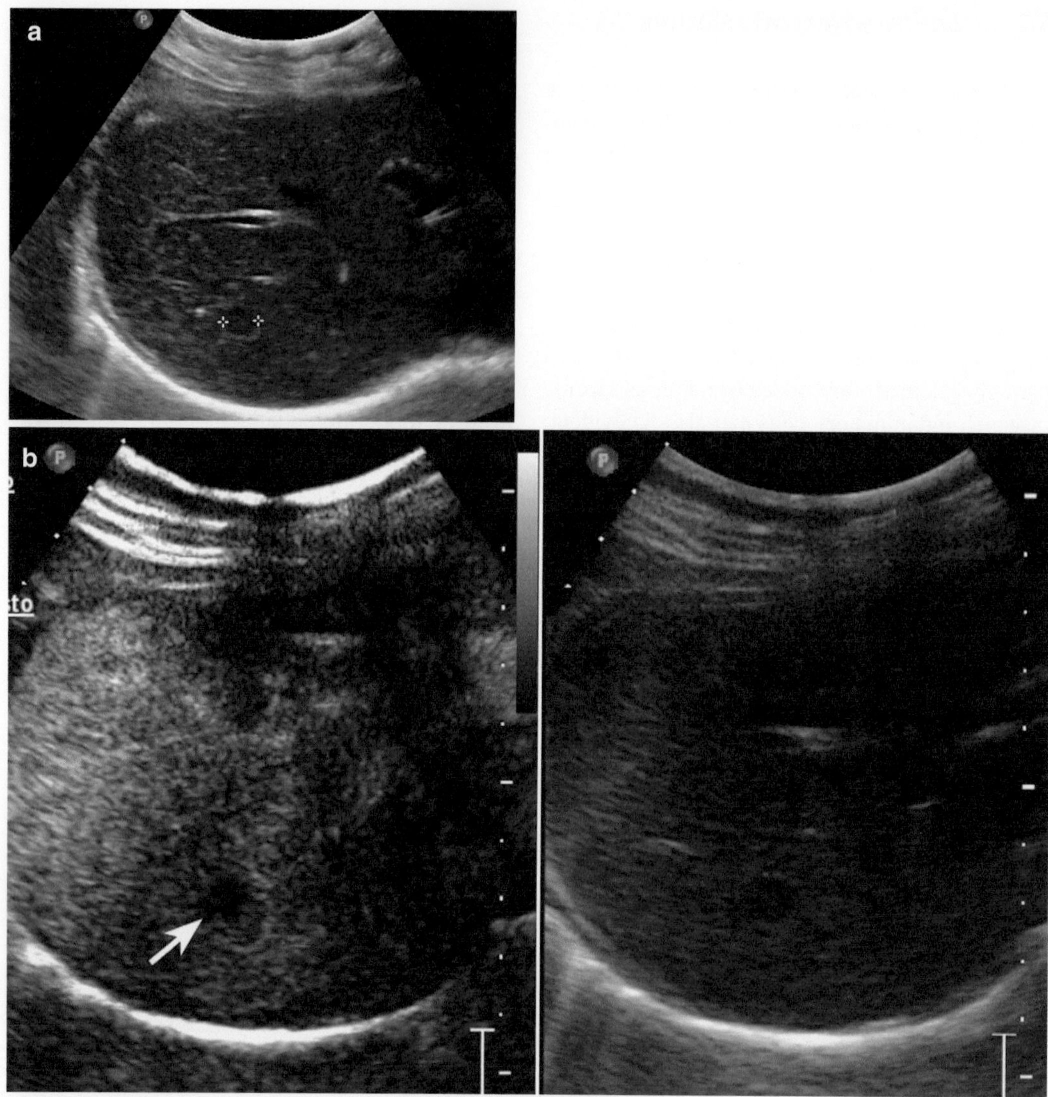

Fig. 5.2 Solitary necrotic nodule in a 66-year-old woman. (**a**) Oblique ascending right subcostal baseline image reveals a small homogeneous hypoechoic lesion sized 1 cm in the VII hepatic segment (calipers). (**b–d**) At CEUS, the lesion presents hypoechoic aspect throughout the vascular study (*arrows*)

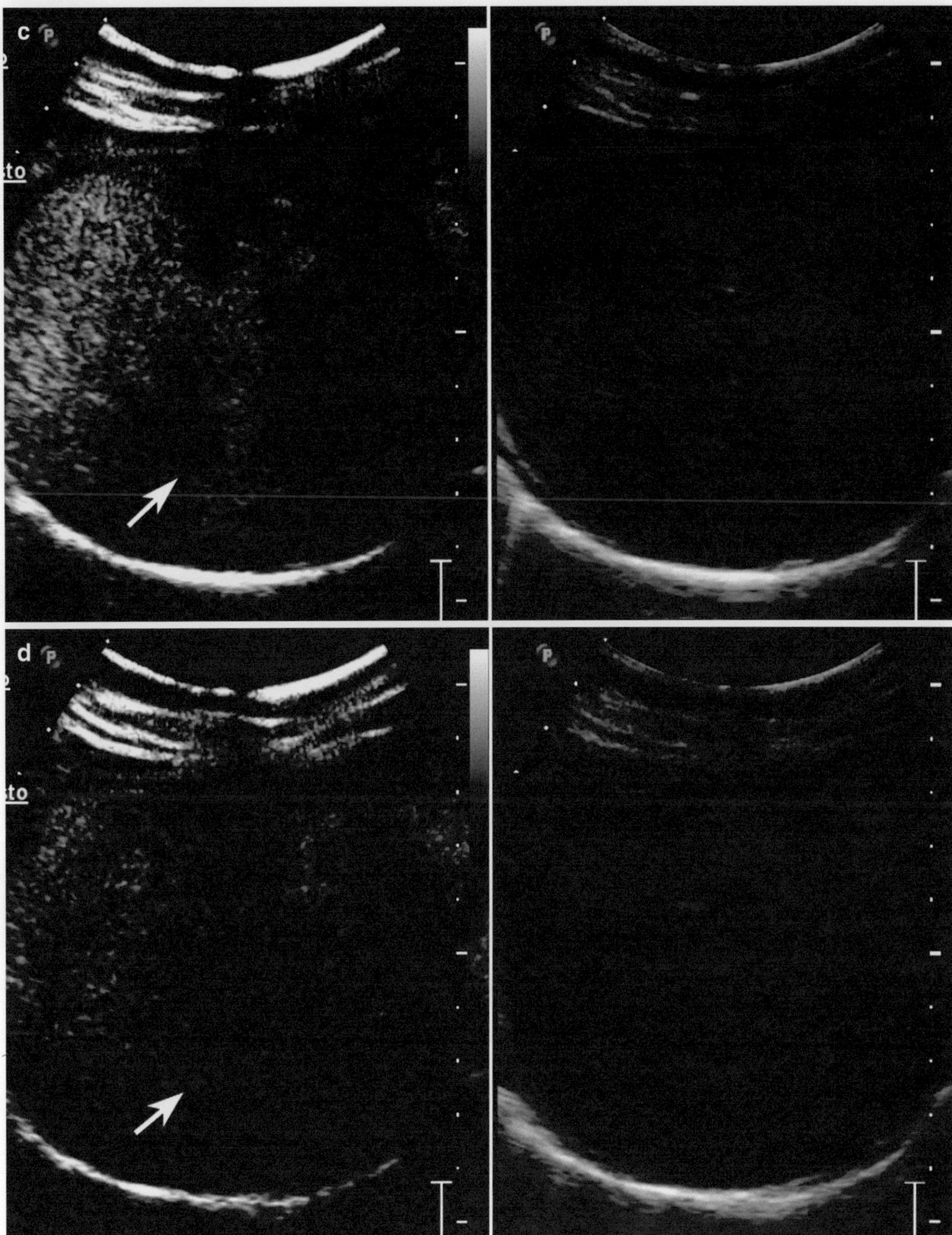

Fig. 5.2 (continued)

5.3   Inflammatory Pseudotumor

The inflammatory pseudotumor (IP) is a benign rare lesion characterized by chronic infiltration of inflammatory cells and areas of fibrosis. It occurs more frequently in the lung whereas the incidence in the liver is very low (around 0.7 %) [14].

The pathogenesis is not clear. Infectious condition, autoimmune phenomenon, or systemic inflammatory response syndrome have been considered as possible pathogenesis [15]. IP can be associated with abdominal pain, vomiting, fever, weight loss, or increased inflammatory markers often directing toward a cancer diagnosis or be completely asymptomatic [16–18]. The final diagnosis, difficult also by means of CT and MR for the absence of peculiar imaging findings, is often obtained by biopsy or surgical resection [19].

At US, the lesion presents mainly hypoechoic, with well-defined margins and homogeneous or inhomogeneous echotexture due to the presence, in some case, of a central hyperechoic or anechoic portion. Usually at color- and power-Doppler evaluation, vascular signal is absent [20]. At CEUS, different patterns can be observed: (a) the lesion can appear constantly hypoechoic; (b) during the arterial phase, IP can show diffuse homogeneous hyperenhancement, diffuse heterogeneous hyperenhancement, peripheral rim-like enhancement, and isoenhancement appearing mainly hypoechoic during the extended portal-venous phase [21, 22].

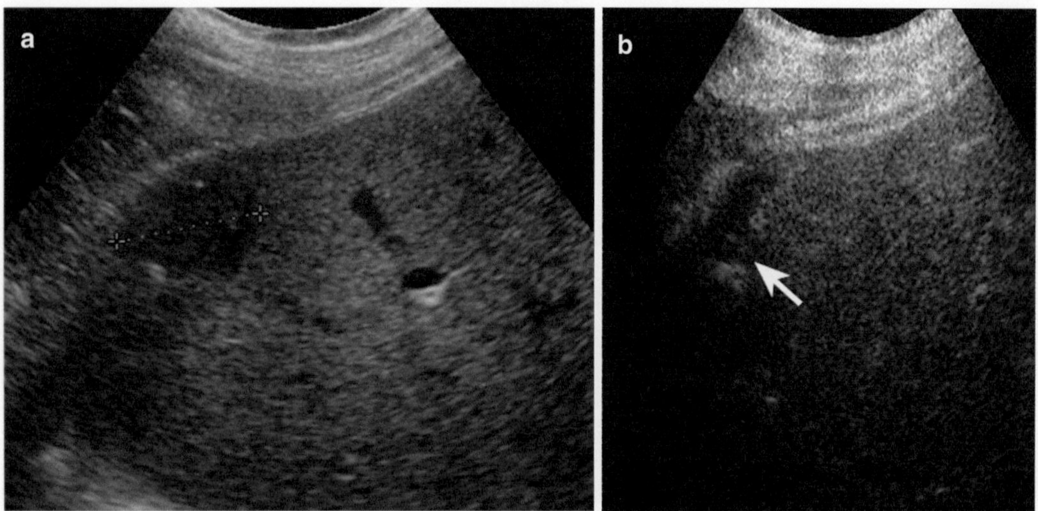

Fig. 5.3 Inflammatory pseudotumor in a 65-year-old man. (**a**) Oblique ascending right subcostal baseline image reveals a hypoechoic lesion sized 3 cm in the VI hepatic segment (calipers). (**b**) At CEUS, peripheral enhancing vessels are appreciable in the portal-venous phase, but the lesion remains hypoechoic (*arrow*)

5.4 Hemangiopericytoma (Lypomatous Subtype)

Hemangiopericytoma is a rare hypervascular tumor which can develop throughout the body in soft tissue and bone, arising from primitive mesenchimal cells located around the vessels called cells of Zimmerman. Hemangiopericytoma may occur at any age but is most common in fifth and sixth decades with the same frequency in men and women. Usually, this mass arises from the upper and lower extremities but, although infrequently, can develop in the liver too [23, 24].

Most commonly, it shows an intermediate grade of aggressiveness [23]. Anyway, large size (>5 cm), necrosis, increased cellularity, increased mitotic activity (>4 mitotic figures/10 high-powered fields), and cytologic atypia are considered prognostic negative features. So surgical removal is the first treatment with a 5-year survival rate of 70 %. Few data are reported in literature about US, CT, and MR imaging findings. It was described as a large, solitary, well-defined cystic lesion with a hypervascular solid component in the context. Speckled calcifications, necrotic and hemorrhagic areas, and cystic degeneration can occur, but these findings are not sufficient for the final diagnosis that is always surgical [25, 26].

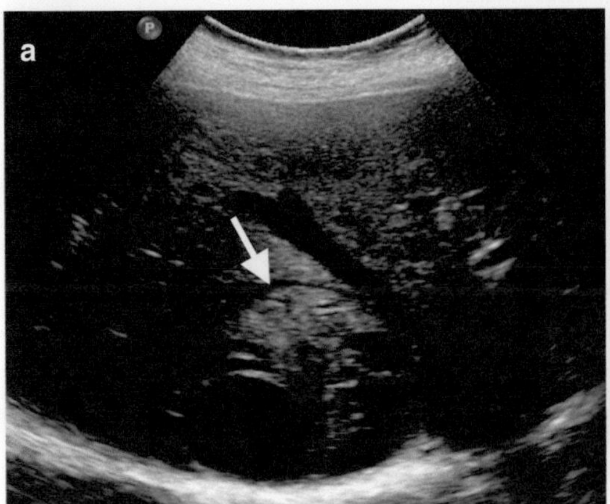
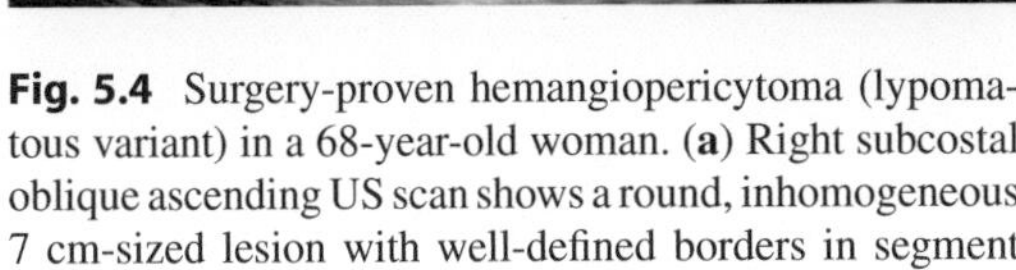
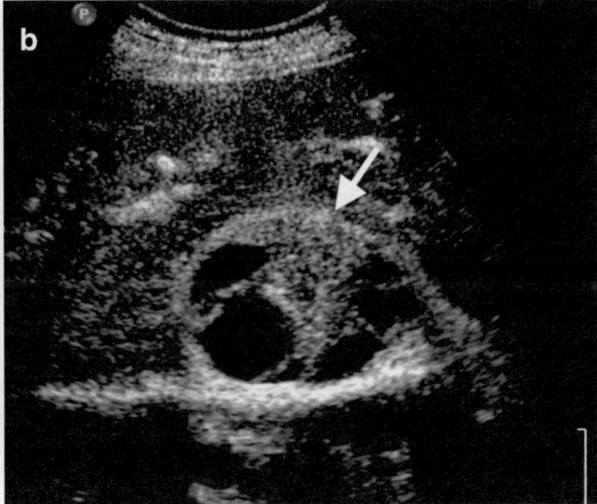

Fig. 5.4 Surgery-proven hemangiopericytoma (lypomatous variant) in a 68-year-old woman. (**a**) Right subcostal oblique ascending US scan shows a round, inhomogeneous 7 cm-sized lesion with well-defined borders in segment VII adjacent to the right hepatic vein (*arrow*). (**b**) After contrast medium injection, the lesion presents inhomogeneous aspect with some fluid areas in the context (*arrow*)

5.5 Extramedullary Intrahepatic Hematopoiesis

The extramedullary hematopoiesis (EH) is considered as a compensatory phenomenon to insufficient production of red blood cells by the bone marrow.

EH involves not only the liver but also other districts such as spleen, lymph nodes, chest, and kidneys. It is associated with severe anemia, congenital hemoglobinopathies, and acquired diseases such as leukemia, lymphoma, or myelofibrosis [27]. At US, the lesion shows well-defined margins, hypoechoic or hyperechoic appearance, and homogeneous or inhomogeneous echotexture due to the presence or not of fatty content [28]. Color Doppler can depict intralesional arterial vascularization [27, 29]. Usually, at CEUS, the lesion appears markedly hypervascular in the arterial phase with sustained but progressively decreasing enhancement in the extended portal venous phase as for focal nodular hyperplasia.

However, the rarity of the lesion and quite unspecific postcontrast findings make necessary biopsy or cytology for the definitive diagnosis in the majority of cases [30].

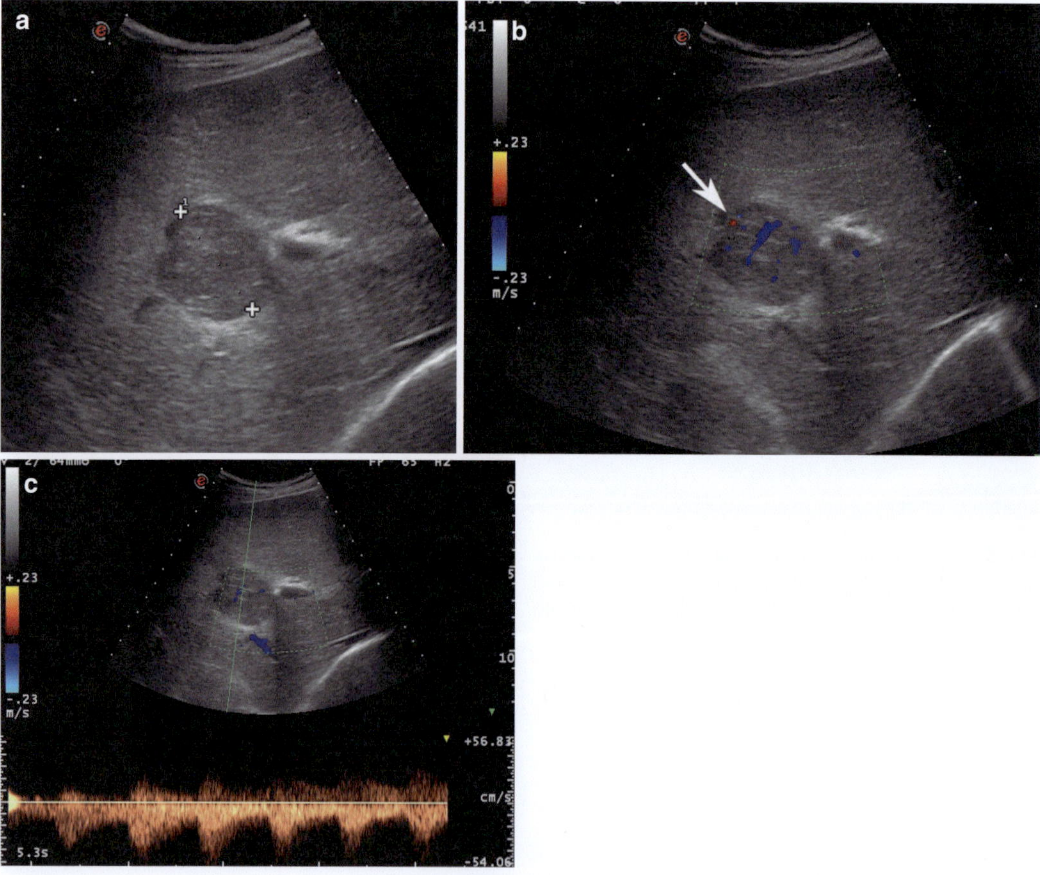

Fig. 5.5 Extramedullary erythropoietic hepatic nodule in a 53-year-old man affected by thalassemia. (**a**) Baseline US image shows a homogeneous hypoechoic lesion sized 4.5 cm in the VI–VII hepatic segment (calipers). (**b, c**) At color-pulsed Doppler evaluation, arterial vascular signal is evident within the mass (*arrow*). (**d**) At CEUS, the lesion appears highly and homogeneously hypervascular in the arterial phase (*arrow*) showing isovascular aspect with respect to the surrounding liver parenchyma during the extended portal-venous phase (**e**)

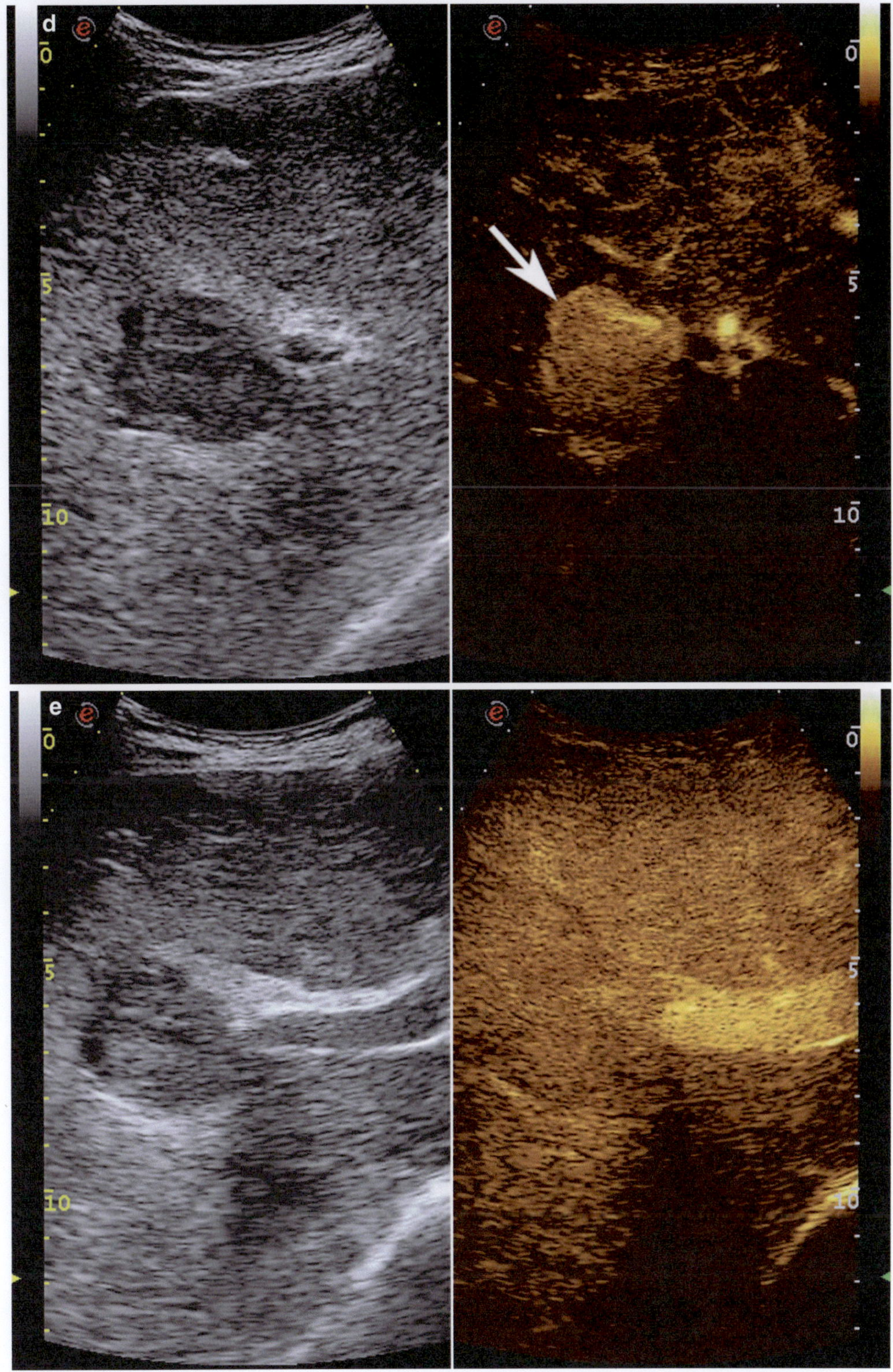

Fig. 5.5 (continued)

5.6   Hepatic Splenosis

Splenosis is considered as the heterotopic auto-transplantation of splenic tissue, more frequently consequence of splenic trauma or surgery in the abdominal, pelvic, or thoracic cavity [31].

It commonly appears on the serosal surfaces of the intestine and mesentery, the omentum, the diaphragm, and the pelvis. In most cases, splenosis is asymptomatic; however, abdominal symptoms such as pain, recurring Felty syndrome, and intestinal obstruction have been reported [32, 33].

Splenic implants are usually multiple and can be localized anywhere in the peritoneal cavity or on the surface of abdominal viscera often mimicking neoplastic lesions [34].

As reported in the only one case report found in literature due to the rarity of the case, hepatic splenosis shows hypoechoic aspect with respect to the surrounding liver parenchyma during the arterial phase and hyperechoic appearance in the extended portal-venous phase [35], whereas the only one case evaluated by CEUS in our department showed homogeneous uptake of contrast medium throughout the vascular study.

Often, the final diagnosis can be reached only by means of percutaneous biopsy in this clinical setting too.

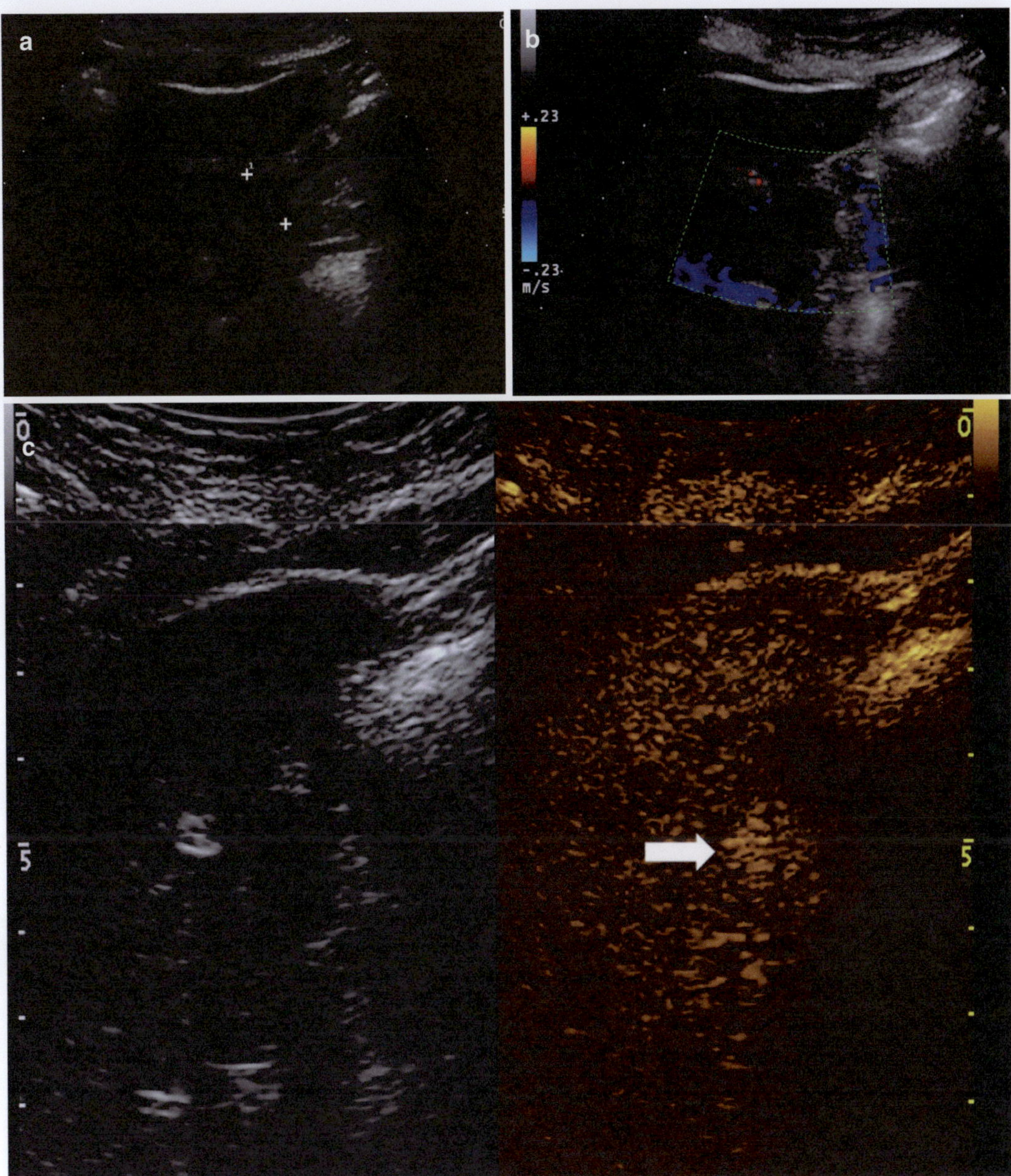

Fig. 5.6 Hepatic splenosis in a 47-year-old woman. (**a**) Sagittal subcostal baseline US image shows a mainly isoechoic lesion sized 1.8 cm in the subcapsular region of the left hepatic lobe (calipers). (**b**) The lesion does not present any vascular signal at color-Doppler evaluation. (**c**) At CEUS, the lesion shows homogeneous uptake of contrast medium (*arrow*)

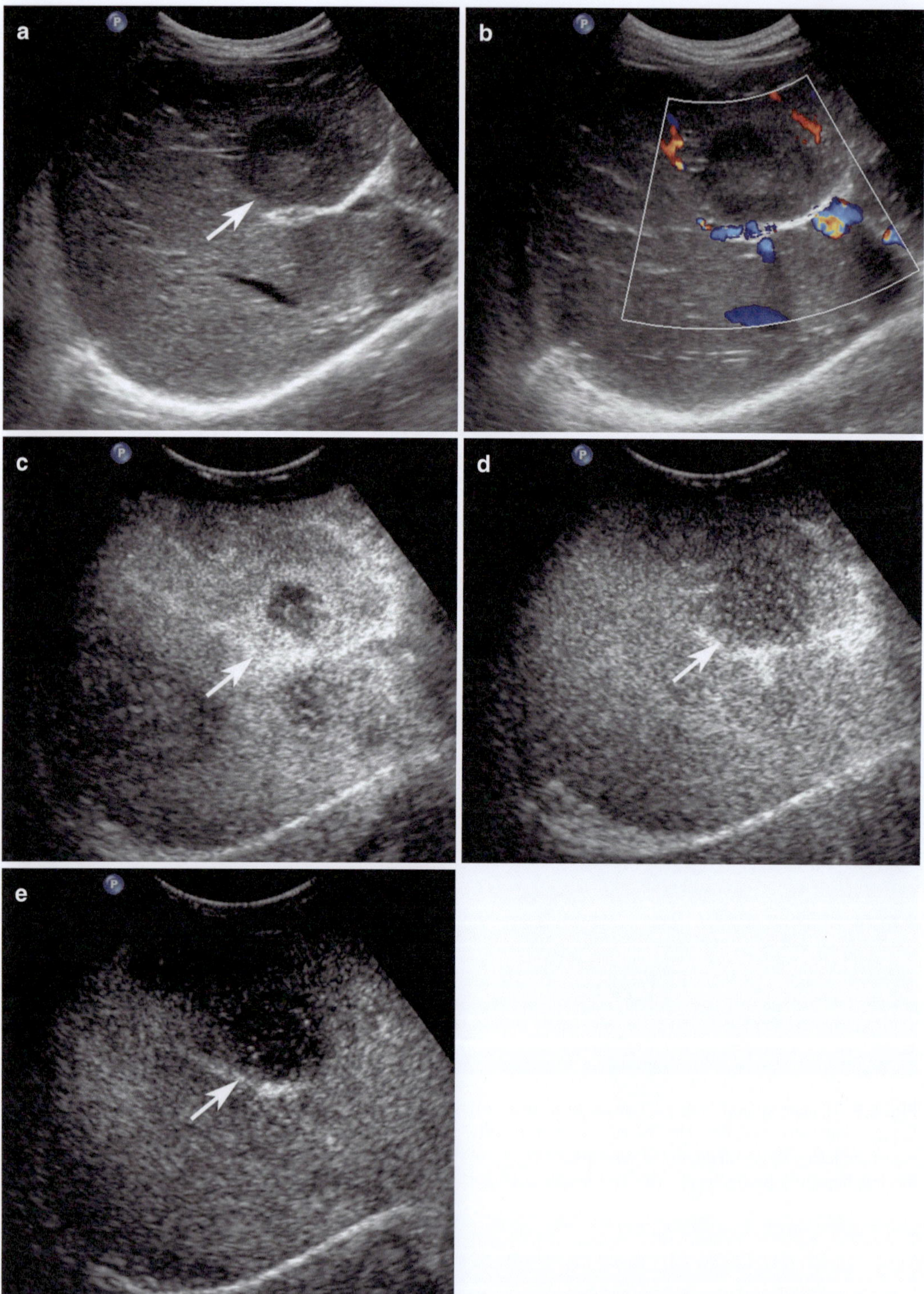

Fig. 5.7 Epithelioid hemangioendothelioma in a 45-year-old woman. (**a**) Oblique ascending right subcostal baseline image reveals an inhomogeneous hypoechoic lesion sized 4.2 cm in the V hepatic segment adjacent to the portal vein (*arrow*). (**b**) The lesion does not show any vascular signal at color-Doppler evaluation. (**c**) In the arterial phase, the lesion appears inhomogeneously hypervascular (*arrow*). (**d**, **e**) In portal-venous and late phases, the lesion shows a progressive washout and appears mainly hypoechoic with respect to the surrounding hepatic parenchyma (*arrows*)

5.7 Epithelioid Hemangioendothelioma

Epithelioid hemangioendothelioma is a rare, low to intermediate grade malignant tumour arising in soft tissues, liver, lung, bone, and spleen. It typically occurs in the 20–40 age range with a female predominance. US depicts lesions that are predominantly hypoechoic but with mixed echotexture ("target" aspect) or predominantly hyperechoic too. CT and MR findings suggestive for hepatic epithelioid hemangioendothelioma include multiple lesions – that can coalesce (diffuse subtype) – mainly located in subcapsular region, in both hepatic lobes with halo or target enhancement patterns in larger lesions Capsular retraction and calcifications can be present. The primary treatment is radical hepatic resection or, in the absence of metastases (most commonly in the lungs), even orthotopic liver transplantation [36, 37].

References

Angiomyolipoma

1. Nonomura A, Enomoto Y, Takeda M et al (2006) Invasive growth of hepatic angiomyolipoma; a hitherto unreported ominous histological feature. Histopathology 48(7):831–835
2. Bartolotta TV, Runza G, Minervini M et al (2003) Hepatic angiomyolipoma: contrast-enhanced US pulse inversion in a case. Radiol Med 105(5–6): 514–518
3. Tajima S, Suzuki A, Suzumura K (2014) Ruptured hepatic epithelioid angiomyolipoma: a case report and literature review. Case Rep Oncol 7(2):369–375
4. Wang B, Ye Z, Chen Y, Zhao Q, Huang M, Chen F et al (2015) Hepatic angiomyolipomas: ultrasonic characteristics of 25 patients from a single center. Ultrasound Med Biol 41(2):393–400
5. Zhong DR, Ji XL (2000) Hepatic angiomyolipoma-misdiagnosis as hepatocellular carcinoma: a report of 14 cases. World J Gastroenterol 6:608–612
6. Wang CP, Li HY, Wang H, Guo XD, Liu CC, Liu SH (2014) Hepatic angiomyolipoma mimicking hepatocellular carcinoma: magnetic resonance imaging and clinical pathological characteristics in 9 cases. Medicine (Baltimore) 93(28):e194

Solitary Necrotic Nodule

7. De Luca M, Louis B, Formisano C et al (2000) Solitary necrotic nodule of the liver misinterpreted as malignant lesion: considerations on two cases. J Surg Oncol 74(3):219–222
8. Yoon KH, Yun KJ, Lee JM et al (2000) Solitary necrotic nodules of the liver mimicking hepatic metastasis: report of two cases. Korean J Radiol 1(3):165–168
9. Colagrande S, Politi LS, Messerini L et al (2003) Solitary necrotic nodule of the liver: imaging and correlation with pathologic features. Abdom Imaging 28:41–44
10. Wang LX, Liu K, Lin GW, Zhai RY (2012) Solitary necrotic nodules of the liver: histology and diagnosis with CT and MRI. Hepat Mon 12(8):e6212
11. Koea J, Taylor G, Miller M et al (2003) Solitary necrotic nodule of the liver: a riddle that is difficult to answer. J Gastrointest Surg 7(5):627–630
12. Iwase K, Higaki J, Yoon HE et al (2002) Solitary necrotic nodule of the liver. J Hepatobiliary Pancreat Surg 9(1):120–124
13. Wang Y, Yu X, Tang J, Li H, Liu L, Gao Y (2007) Solitary necrotic nodule of the liver: contrast-enhanced sonography. J Clin Ultrasound 35(4): 177–181

Inflammatory Pseudotumor

14. Park JY, Choi MS, Lim YS, Park JW, Kim SU, Min YW et al (2014) Clinical features, image findings, and prognosis of inflammatory pseudotumor of the liver: a multicenter experience of 45 cases. Gut Liver 8(1):58–63
15. Locke JE, Choti MA, Torbenson MS et al (2005) Inflammatory pseudotumor of the liver. J Hepatobiliary Pancreat Surg 12(4):314–316
16. Yoon KH, Ha HK, Lee JS et al (1999) Inflammatory pseudotumor of the liver in patients with recurrent pyogenic cholangitis: CT-histopathologic correlation. Radiology 211(2):373–379
17. Park KS, Jang BK, Chung W et al (2006) Inflammatory pseudotumor of liver: a clinical review of 15 cases. Korean J Hepatol 12(3):429–438
18. Schuessler G, Fellbaum C, Fauth F et al (2006) The inflammatory pseudotumor – an unusual liver tumor. Ultraschall Med 27(3):273–279
19. Saito K, Kotake F, Ito N et al (2002) Inflammatory pseudotumor of the liver in a patient with rectal cancer: a case report. Eur Radiol 12(10):2484–2487
20. Lim JH, Lee JH (1995) Inflammatory pseudotumor of the liver. Ultrasound and CT features. Clin Imaging 19(1):43–46

21. Koide H, Sato K, Fukusato T et al (2006) Spontaneous regression of hepatic inflammatory pseudotumor with primary biliary cirrhosis: a case report and literature review. World J Gastroenterol 12(10):1645–1648
22. Kong WT, Wang WP, Cai H, Huang BJ, Ding H, Mao F (2014) The analysis of enhancement pattern of hepatic inflammatory pseudotumor on contrast-enhanced ultrasound. Abdom Imaging 39(1):168–174

Hemangiopericytoma (Lypomatous Subtype)

23. Vilanova J, Barcelò J, Smirniotopoulos J et al (2004) Hemangioma from head to toe: MR imaging with pathologic correlation. Radiographics 24:367–385
24. Bokshan SL, Doyle M, Becker N, Nalbantoglu I, Chapman WC (2012) Hepatic hemangiopericytoma/solitary fibrous tumor: a review of our current understanding and case study. J Gastrointest Surg 16(11):2170–2176
25. Cheng NY, Chen RC, Chen TY, Tu HY (2008) Contrast-enhanced ultrasonography of hepatic metastasis of hemangiopericytoma. J Ultrasound Med 27(4):667–671
26. Aliberti C, Benea G, Kopf B, De Giorgi U (2006) Hepatic metastases of hemangiopericytoma: contrast-enhanced MRI, contrast-enhanced ultrasonography and angiography findings. Cancer Imaging 6:56–59

Extramedullary Intrahepatic Hematopopiesis

27. Aytac S, Fitoz S, Akyar S et al (1999) Focal intrahepatic extramedullary hematopoiesis: color Doppler US and CT findings. Abdom Imaging 24:366–368
28. Gupta P, Naran A, Auh YH et al (2004) Focal intrahepatic extramedullary hematopoiesis presenting as fatty lesions. AJR Am J Roentgenol 182(4):1031–1032
29. Wong Y, Chen F, Tai KS et al (1999) Imaging features of focal intrahepatic extramedullary hematopoiesis. J Radiol Br 72:906–910
30. Quaia E (2007) Mezzi di contrasto in ecografia. Applicazioni addominali. Springer, Milan

Hepatic Splenosis

31. Tsitouridis I, Michaelides M, Sotiriadis C, Arvaniti M (2010) CT and MRI of intraperitoneal splenosis. Diagn Interv Radiol 16(2):145–149
32. Hovius JW, Verberne HJ, Bennink RJ, Blok WL (2010) The (re)generation of splenic tissue. BMJ Case Rep 2010. pii:bcr0320102833. doi:10.1136/bcr.03.2010.2833
33. Choi GH, Ju MK, Kim JY, Kang CM, Kim KS, Choi JS et al (2008) Hepatic splenosis preoperatively diagnosed as hepatocellular carcinoma in a patient with chronic hepatitis B: a case report. J Korean Med Sci 23(2):336–341
34. Imbriaco M, Camera L, Manciuria A, Salvatore M (2008) A case of multiple intra-abdominal splenosis with computed tomography and magnetic resonance imaging correlative findings. World J Gastroenterol 14(9):1453–1455
35. Ferraioli G, Di Sarno A, Coppola C, Giorgio A (2006) Contrast-enhanced low-mechanical-index ultrasonography in hepatic splenosis. J Ultrasound Med 25(1):133–136

Epithelioid Hemangioendothelioma

36. Earnest F, Johnson CD (2006) Case 96: Hepatic epithelioid hemangioendothelioma. Radiology 240:295–298
37. Mermuys K, Vanhoenacker PK, Roskams T, D'Haenens P, Van Hoe L (2004) Epithelioid hemangioendothelioma of the liver: radiologic-pathologic correlation. Abdom Imaging 29:221–223

During the last decades, invasive and semi-invasive locoregional treatments have been developed and improved for the treatment of primary and secondary hepatic tumors. Efficacy of these therapies is usually monitored by means of contrast-enhanced CT and MR. The goal is documenting the lack of vascularization in the treated area and early detection of tumor recurrence allowing further treatments and thus increasing life expectancy.

CT and MR represent the gold standard for the evaluation of the therapeutic response after local treatments. But, as already confirmed by several studies, CEUS represents a reliable alternative technique since it allows the study in real time of microcirculation useful for an early detection of viable tissue [1]. Moreover, it represents a useful tool before locoregional treatments in order to better define lesion's margins and for an adequate radiofrequency needle placement [2].

Also at CEUS, a complete response is considered achieved when there is no enhancing portion within or at the periphery of the treated area during the hepatic arterial phase [3, 4]. Residual unablated tumor is defined as a portion of treated HCC showing persistent hypervascularity in the arterial phase, usually appearing as an irregular peripheral-enhancing focus in the treated zone. When viable tumoral tissue, enhancing at arterial phase acquisition, is detected within the edge of a treated nodule, the pattern is called "in-growth" whereas when it is depicted around a necrotic treated nodule and in continuity with its border, the term "out-growth" could be used.

Immediately and up to 3 months after the treatment, a quite uniform and relatively thin (usually 4–5 to 7–8 mm thick) peripheral rim of contrast enhancement surrounding the treated zone can be evident as a local response to thermal damage due to benign reactive hyperemia [5]. The rim of hyperemia may sometimes be difficult to differentiate from actual residual tumor, but usually it is thin, completely surrounding the treated area, and disappears over time. Another area presenting as transient hypervascular area in the arterial phase may be related to the presence of arteriovenous shunting and may also lead to misinterpretation. This perfusion alteration becomes isoechoic to the surrounding liver parenchyma in the extended portal venous phase and the characteristics of a peripheral-based wedge-shaped pattern are helpful to differentiate this entity from residual tumor. The term tumor progression usually refers to the presence of growing enhancing tumors at the periphery of treated area at CEUS later than 1-month follow-up but with no evidence of residual tumor in the previous controls [6, 7].

© Springer International Publishing Switzerland 2015
T.V. Bartolotta et al., *Atlas of Contrast-enhanced Sonography of Focal Liver Lesions*,
DOI 10.1007/978-3-319-17539-3_6

6.1 Locoregional Treatment

6.1.1 RFTA

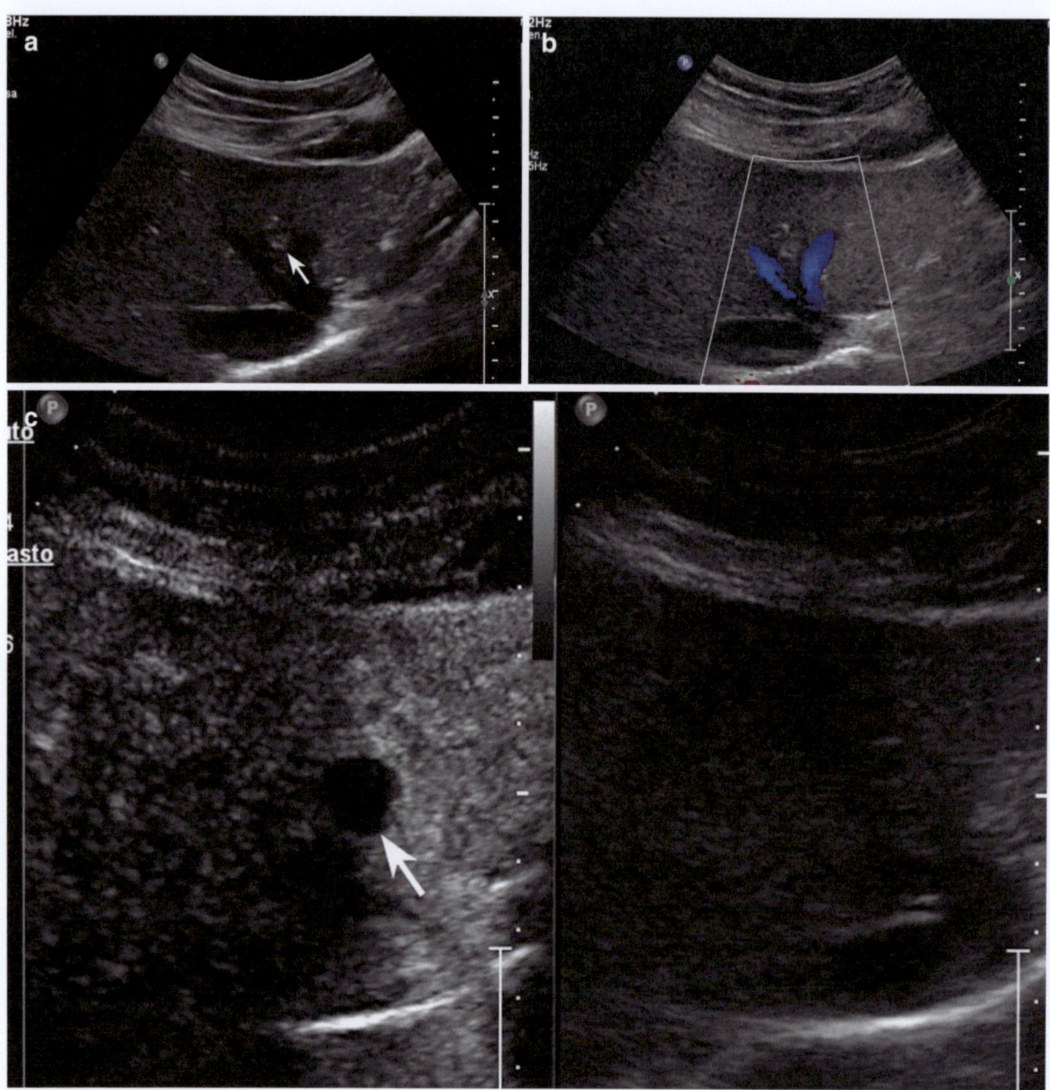

Fig. 6.1 Complete response in RFTA-treated colorectal metastasis in a 55-year-old woman. (**a**) Central subcostal baseline US image shows a 1 cm-sized slightly inhomogeneous hyperechoic area in the IV hepatic segment (*arrow*) without vascularization at color-Doppler evaluation (**b**). At CEUS, the lesion shows lack of contrast enhancement in the arterial (**c**) and extended portal-venous (**d**) phases (*left, arrows*)

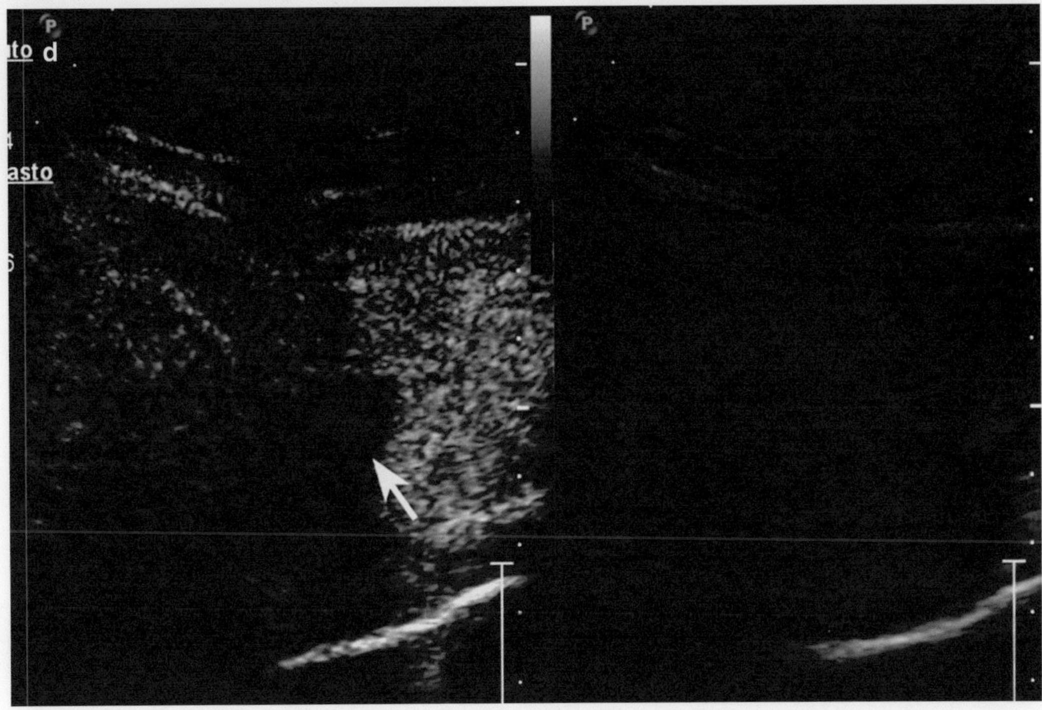

Fig. 6.1 (continued)

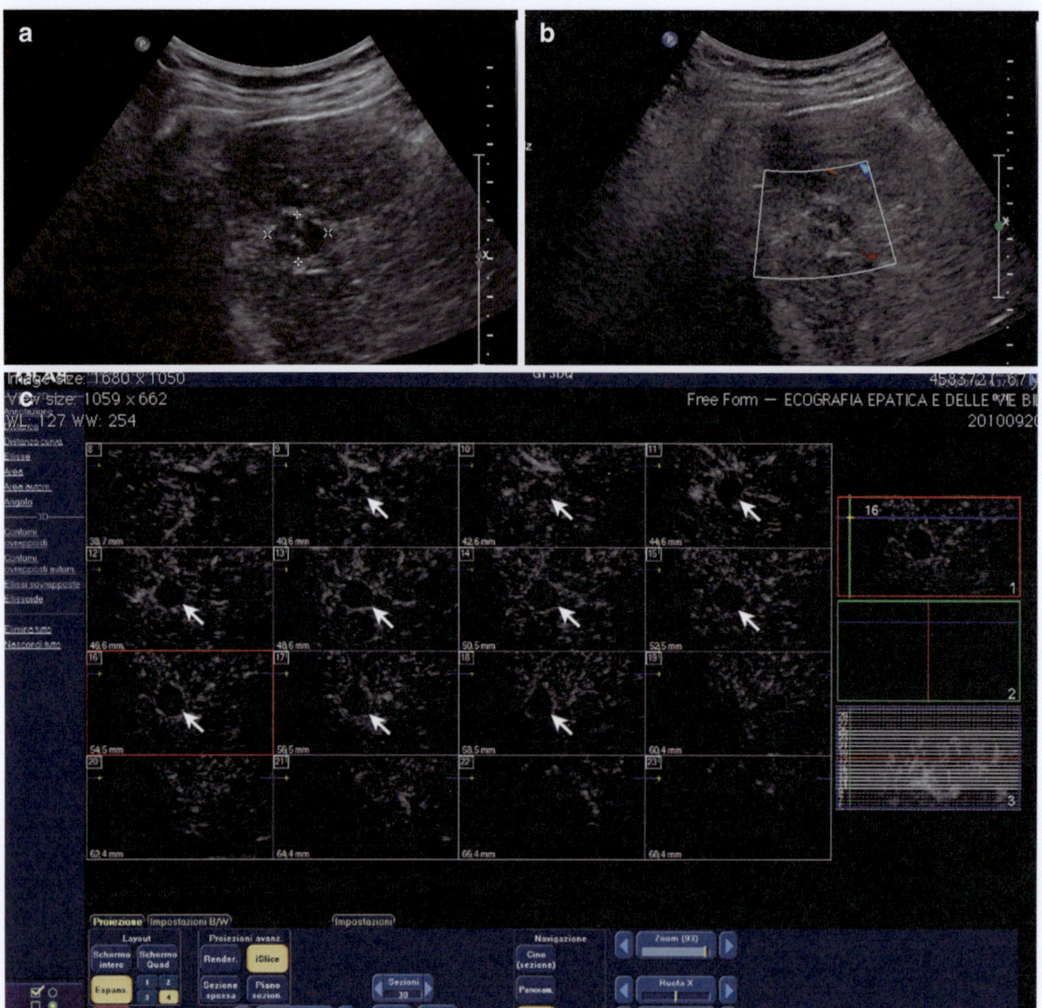

Fig. 6.2 Complete response after RFTA in a 49-year-old man. (**a**) Oblique ascending right subcostal baseline US image shows a 1.7 cm-sized inhomogeneous hypoechoic area in the V hepatic segment (*calipers*) without vascularization at color-Doppler evaluation (**b**); (**c**) At 3D-CEUS, i-Slice reconstruction shows lack of contrast enhancement in each slice during the arterial phase (*arrows*); (**d**) Volumetric reconstruction on three planes shows the entire volume of the treated area

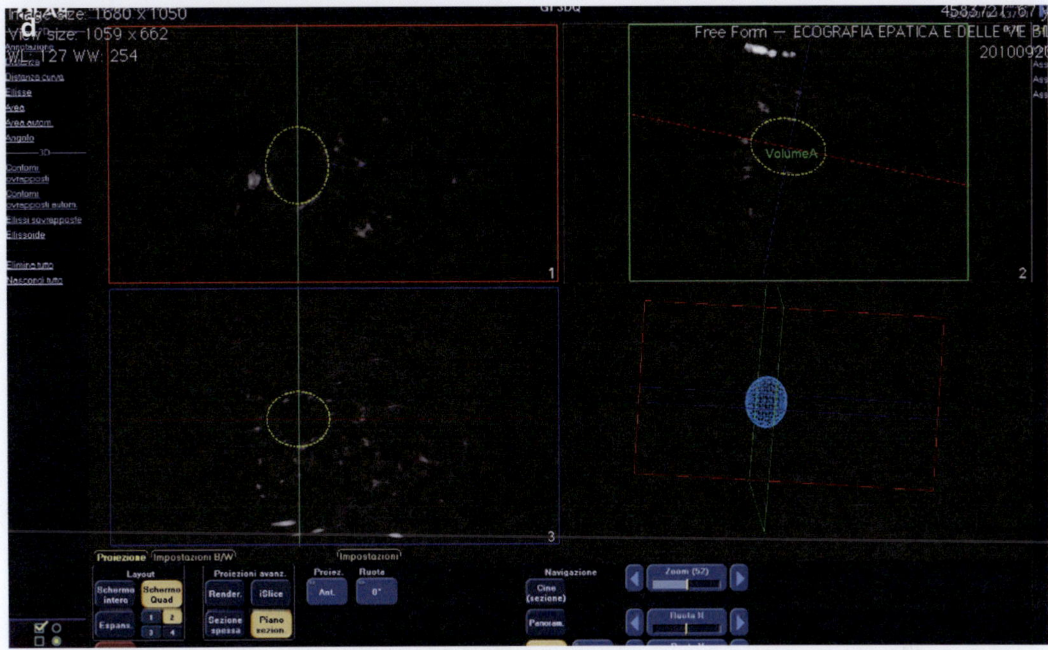

Fig. 6.2 (continued)

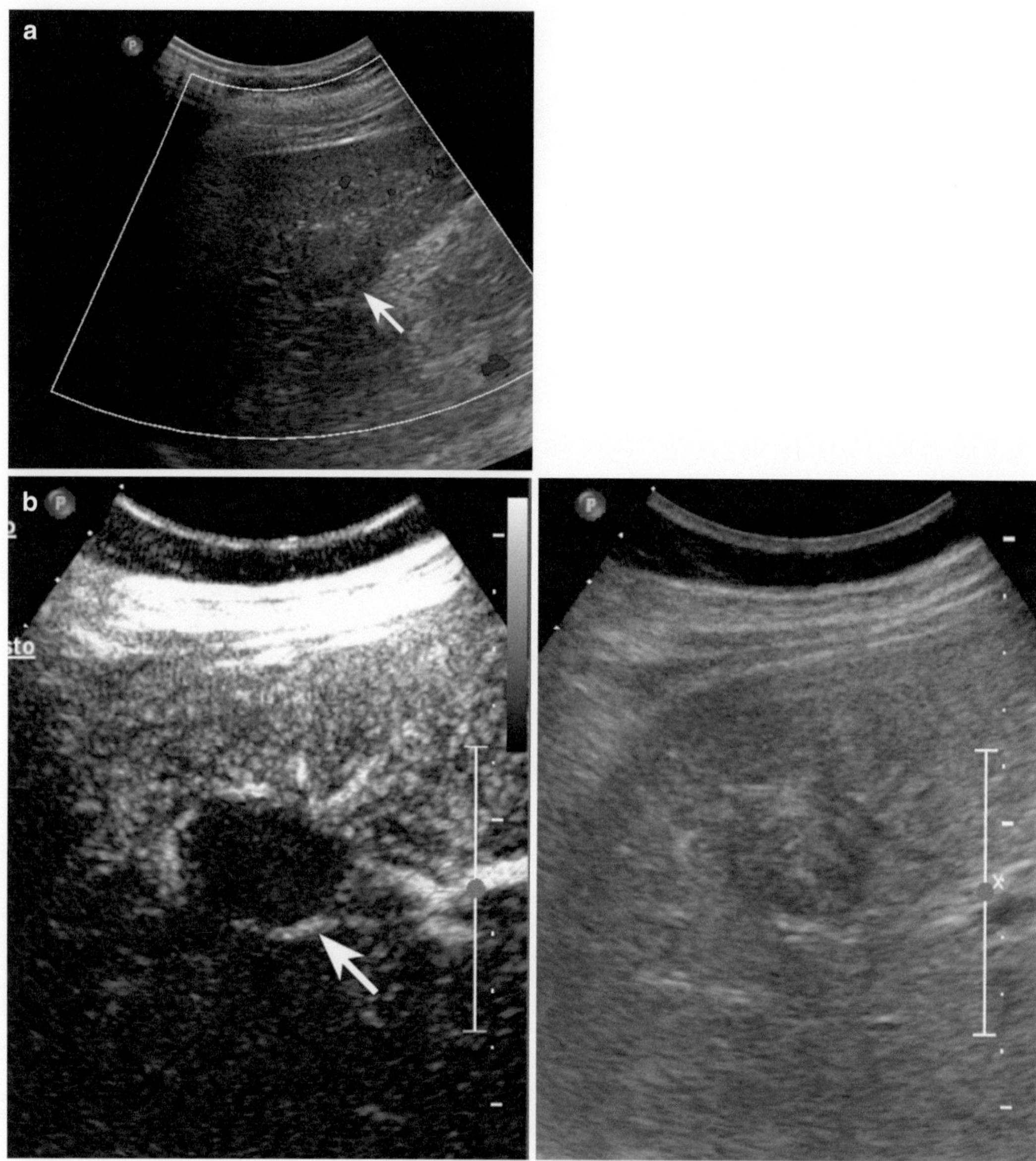

Fig. 6.3 Rim of hyperemia in RFTA-treated HCC in a 63-year-old man. (**a**) Oblique ascending right subcostal image reveals a slightly hypoechoic 3 cm-sized area in the V hepatic segment in the subcapsular region, with absence of vascularization at color-Doppler evaluation (*arrow*). (**b**) At CEUS 1 month after RFA, a thin peripheral rim of contrast enhancement surrounding the ablated zone is evident in the arterial phase (27 s after SonoVue injection) (*left*, *arrow*) and no more appreciable in the remaining portal-venous (**c**) and late phases (**d**) (*arrows*)

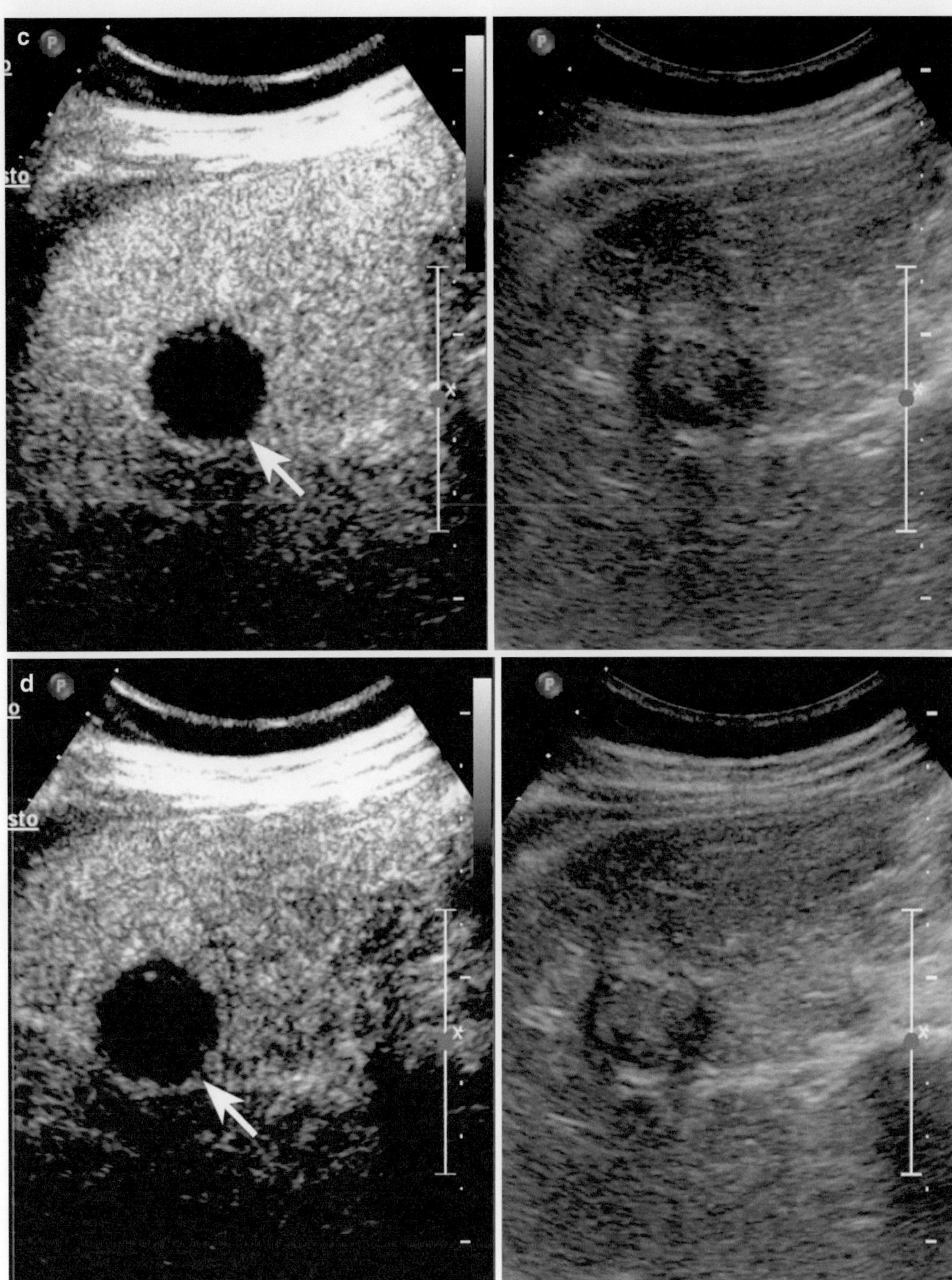

Fig. 6.3 (continued)

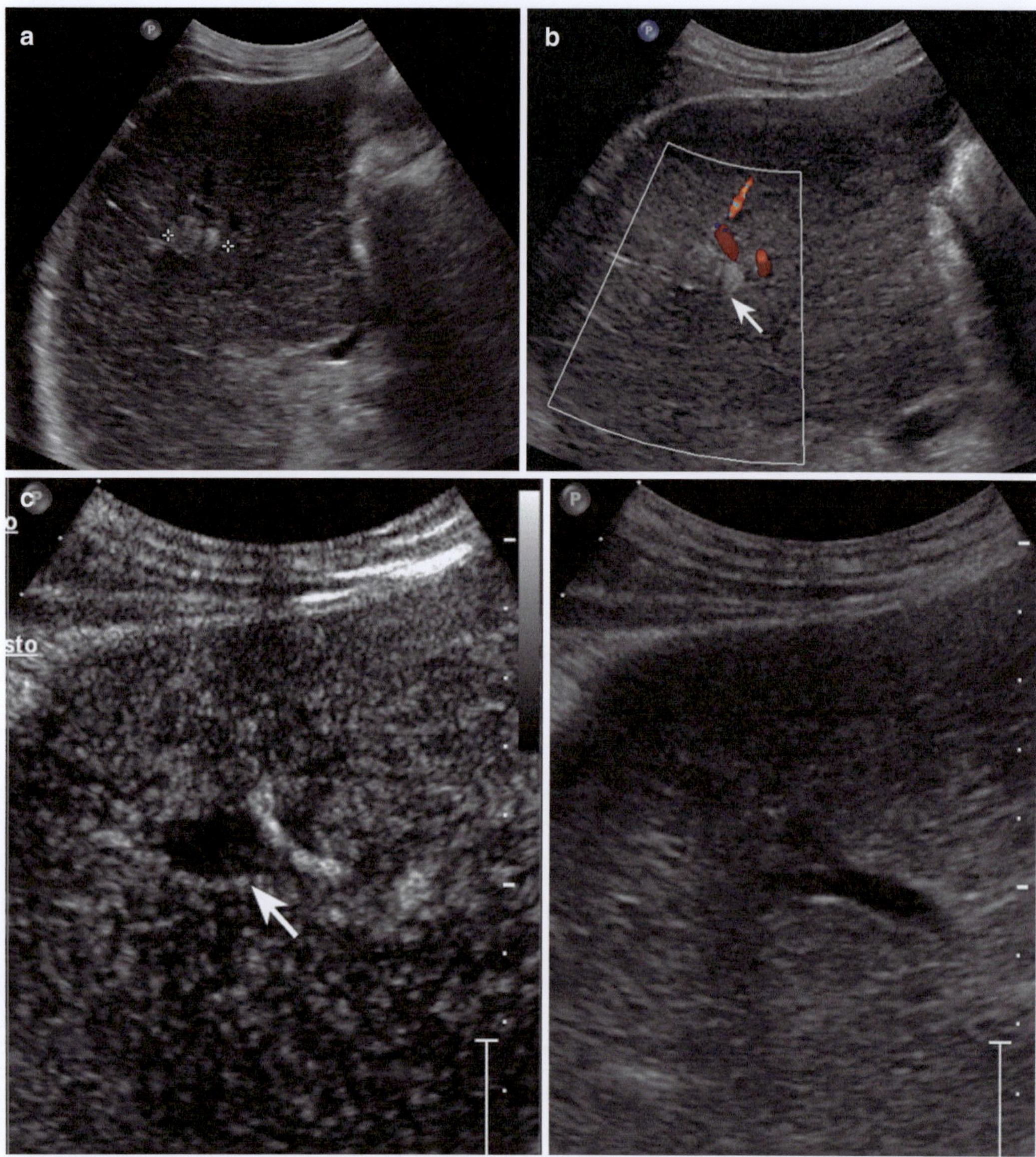

Fig. 6.4 Complete response after RFTA in a 57-year-old man. (**a**) Oblique ascending right subcostal baseline US image shows a 2 cm-sized inhomogeneous hyperechoic area in the V hepatic segment (*calipers*) without vascularization at color-Doppler evaluation (*arrow*) (**b**). (**c**) At CEUS in the arterial phase, the lesion shows lack of contrast enhancement (*left, arrow*); (**d**) 3D i-Slice reconstruction shows the same finding appreciable in each slice (*arrows*); (**e**) Volumetric reconstruction on three planes shows that the treated area has a total volume of 0.71 mL (*arrow*)

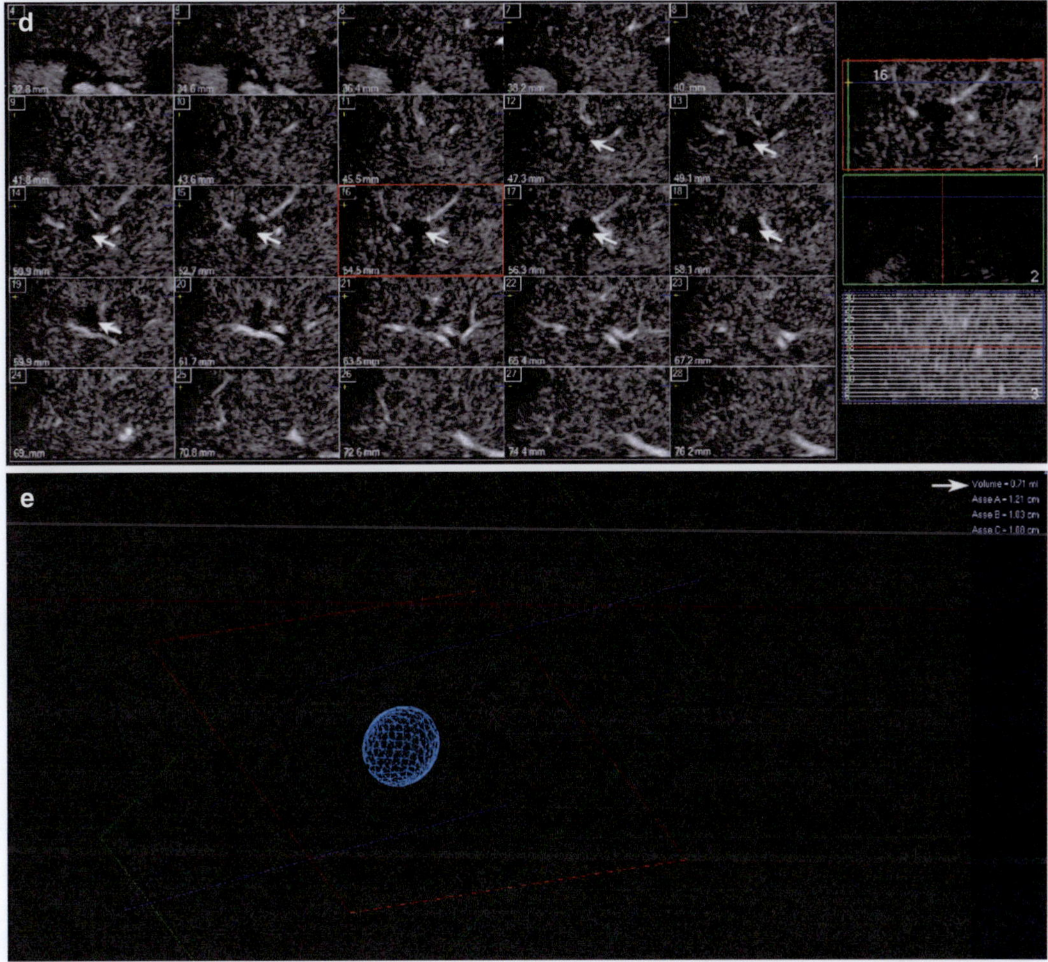

Fig. 6.4 (continued)

6.1.2   TACE

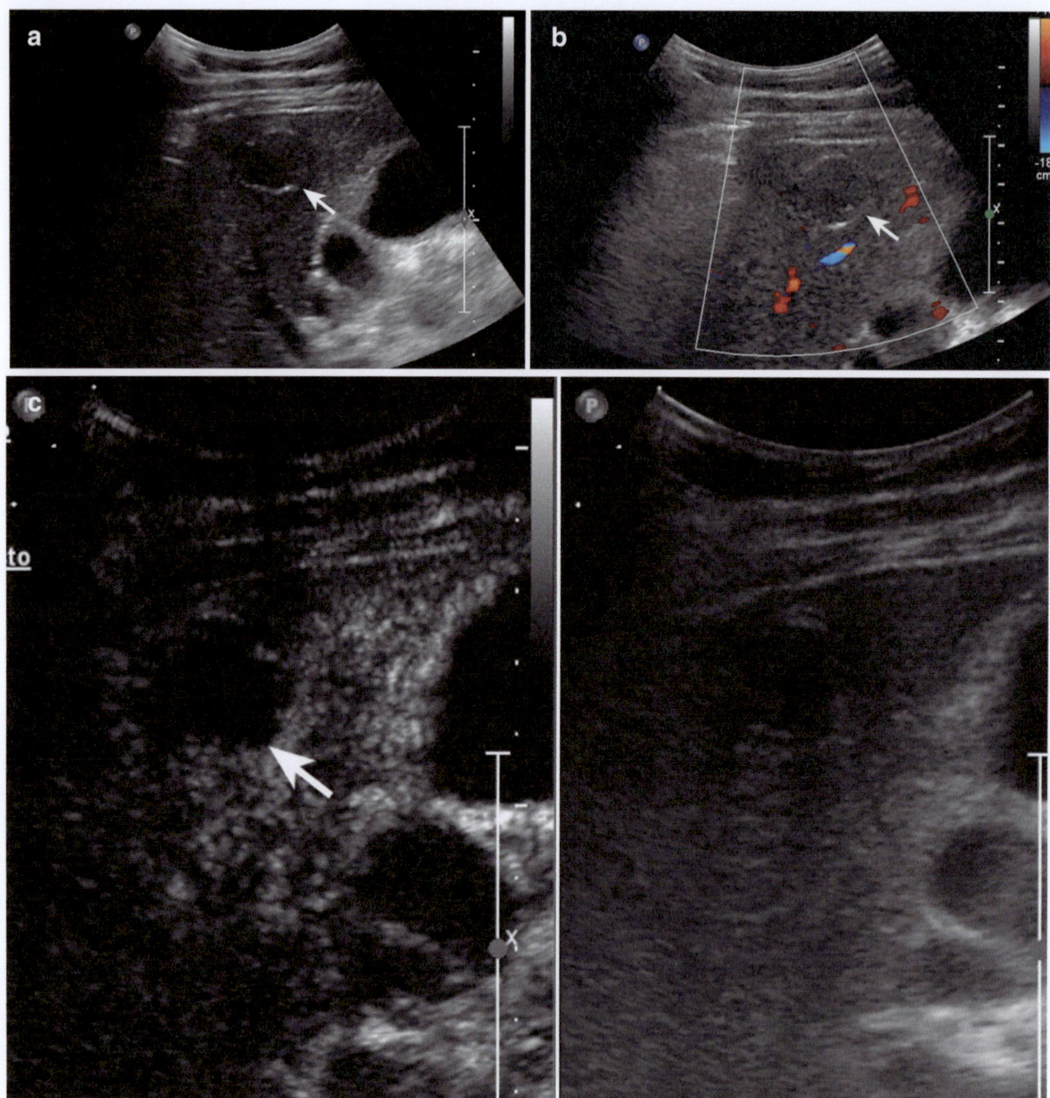

Fig. 6.5 Complete response after TACE in a 55-year-old man. (**a**) Right intercostal baseline US image shows a 2 cm-sized inhomogeneous hypoechoic area in the V hepatic segment without vascularization at color-Doppler evaluation (*arrows*) (**b**); (**c**) At CEUS, the lesion shows lack of contrast enhancement in the arterial phase (*left*, *arrow*)

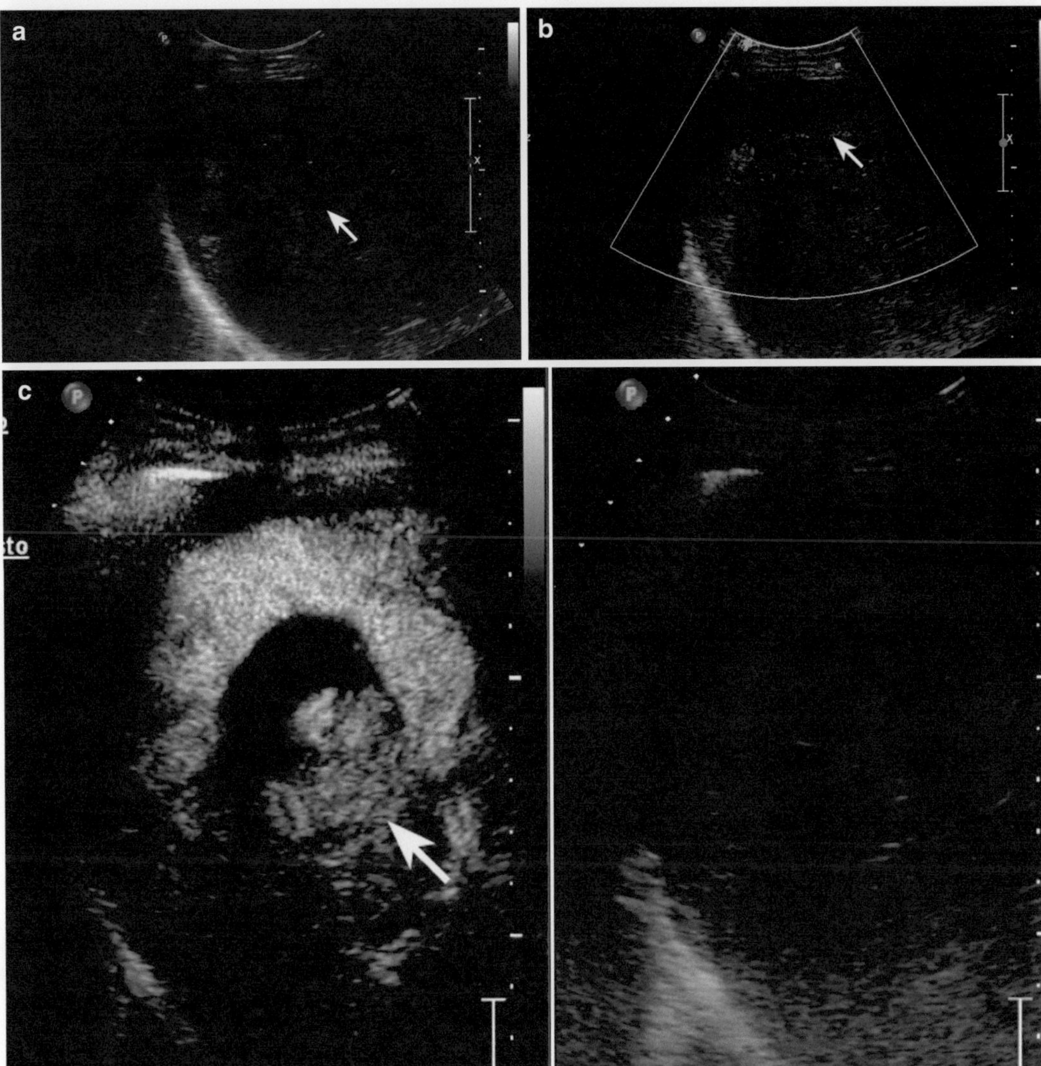

Fig. 6.6 Residual tumor after combined TACE-RFTA treatment in a 52-year-old man. (**a**) Axial baseline image shows a 8.9 cm-sized inhomogeneous hypoechoic area with ill-defined margins and some tiny vascular signal at color-Doppler evaluation (**b**) (*arrows*); (**c**) At CEUS, a highly hypervascular tissue is evident within the treated area in the arterial phase (*arrow*). (**d**) This tissue shows washout in the portal venous phase (*arrow*)

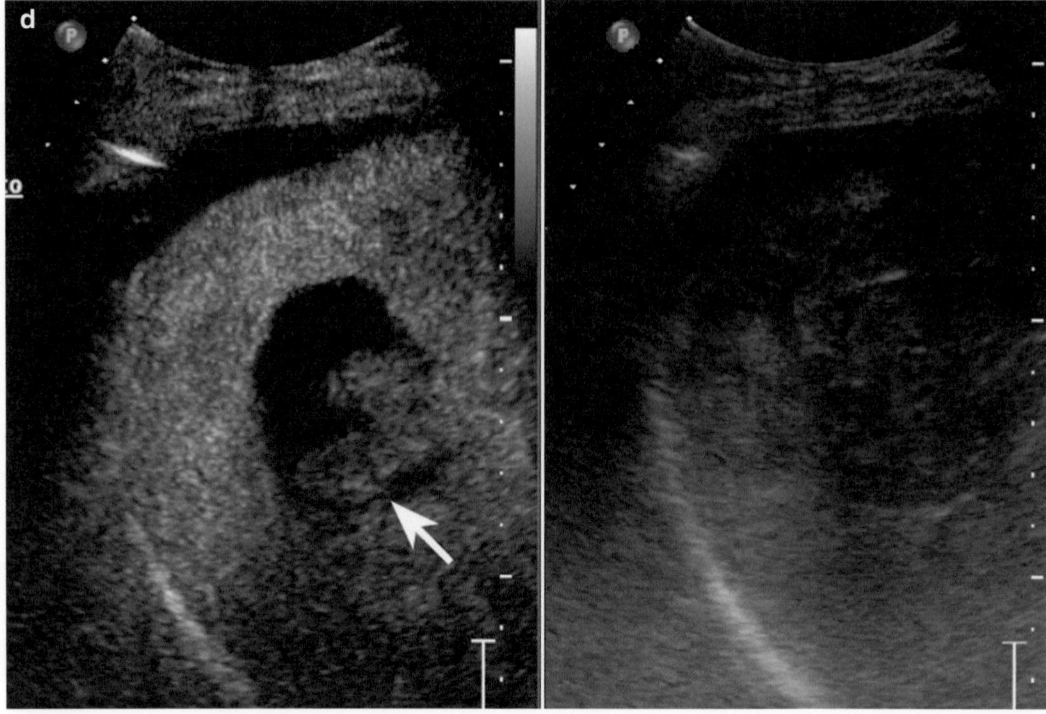

Fig. 6.6 (continued)

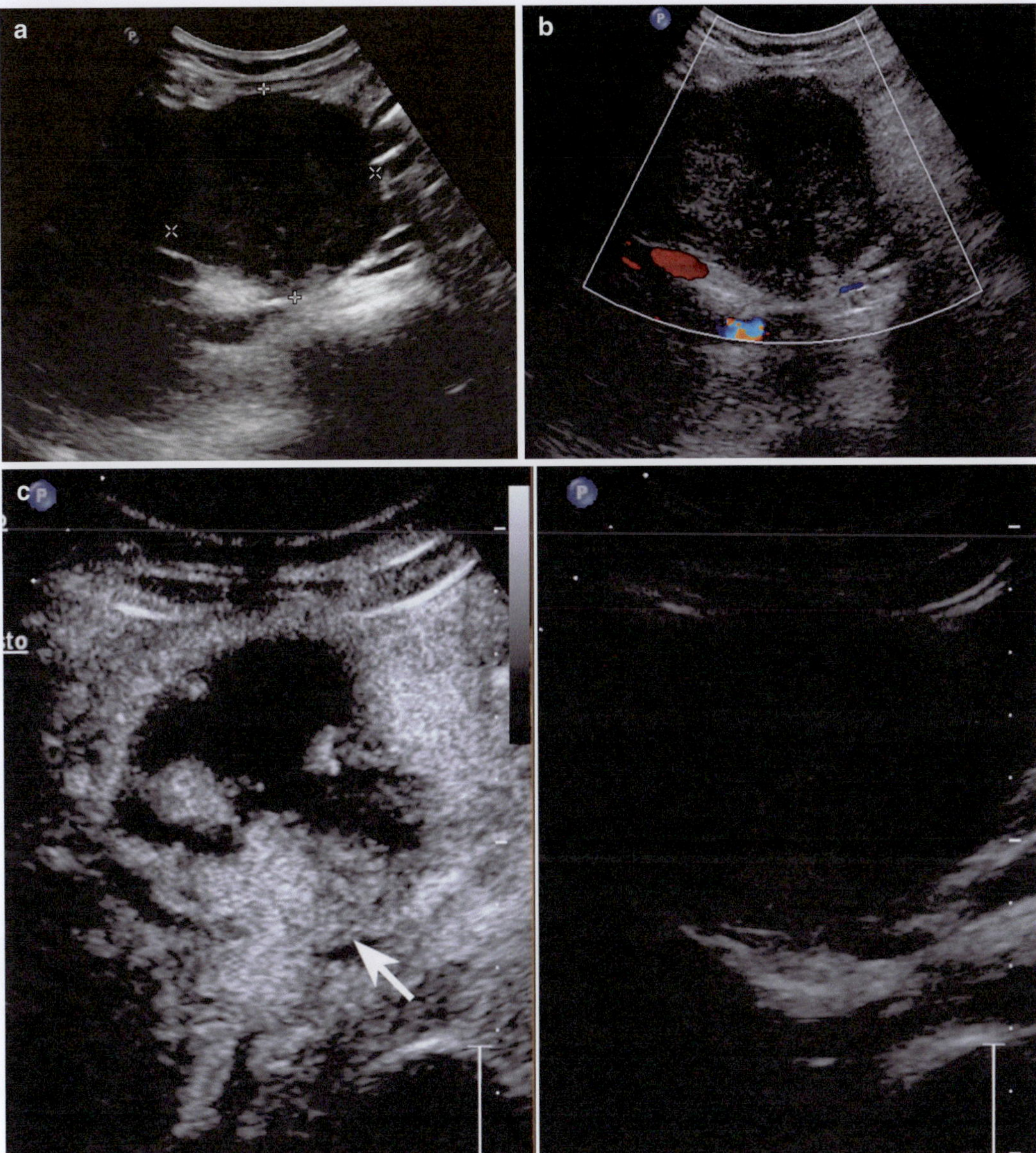

Fig. 6.7 Residual tumor after TACE in a 52-year-old woman. (**a**) Axial baseline US image of the left lobe shows a 6.7 cm-sized inhomogeneous mass (*calipers*) without evident vascular signal at color-Doppler evalua-tion (**b**); (**c**) At CEUS in the arterial phase, a highly hyper-vascular tissue within the treated area is evident (*arrow*) showing wash- out in the remaining vascular phases (**d, e**) (*arrows*)

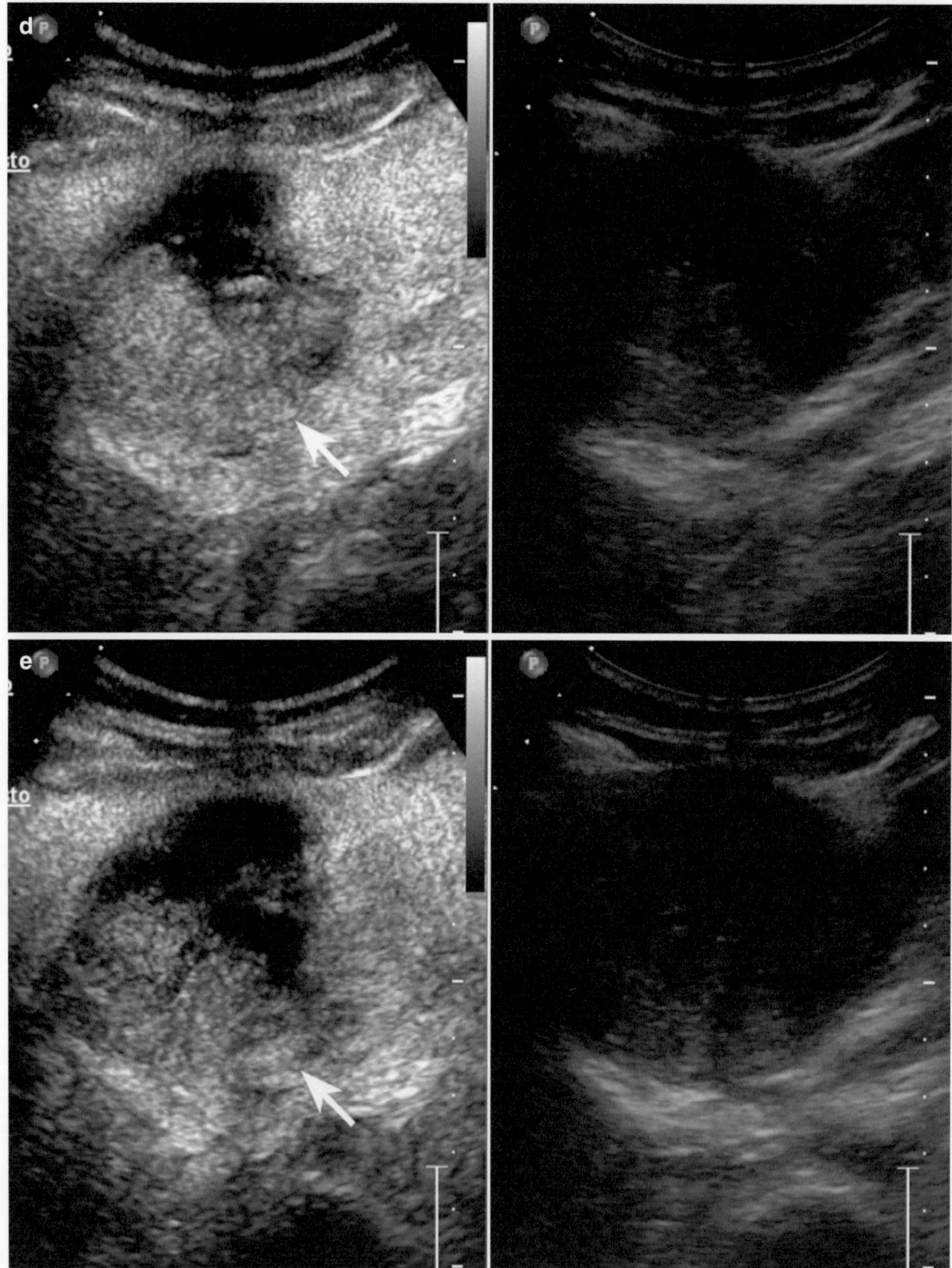

Fig. 6.7 (continued)

6.1.3 Habib Resection

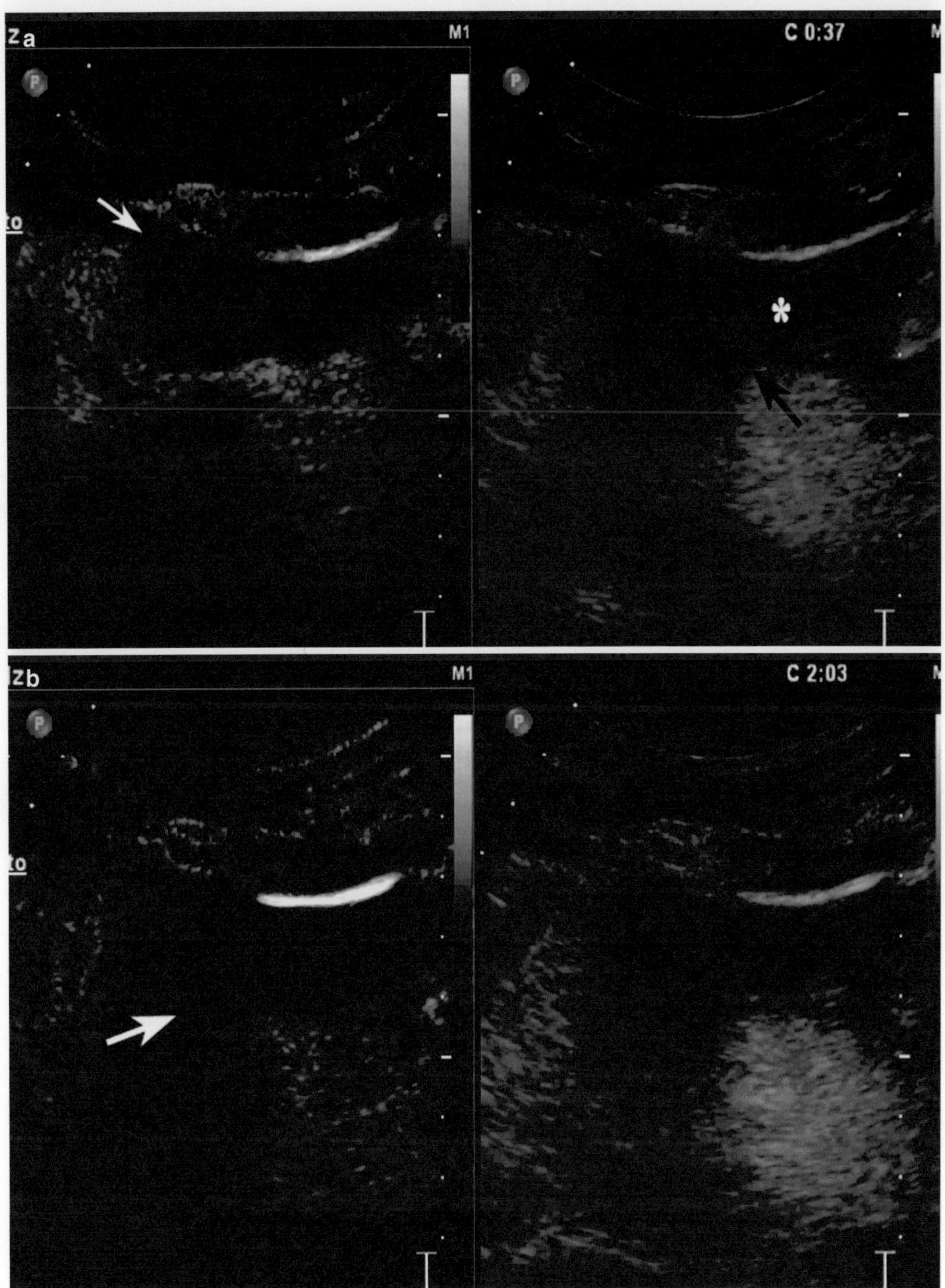

Fig. 6.8 Complete necrosis in a 64-year-old man with hepatocellular carcinoma treated with bipolar radiofrequency electrosurgical device at CEUS follow-up in a 68 year-old man. (**a**) Unenhanced US image demonstrates a hypoechoic peripheral halo (*black arrow*) surrounding a fluid collection (*asterisk*) (*right side*). At CEUS, this area shows lack of contrast enhancement in the arterial phase (*white arrow, left side*) and (**b**) in the extended portal-venous phase (*arrow*)

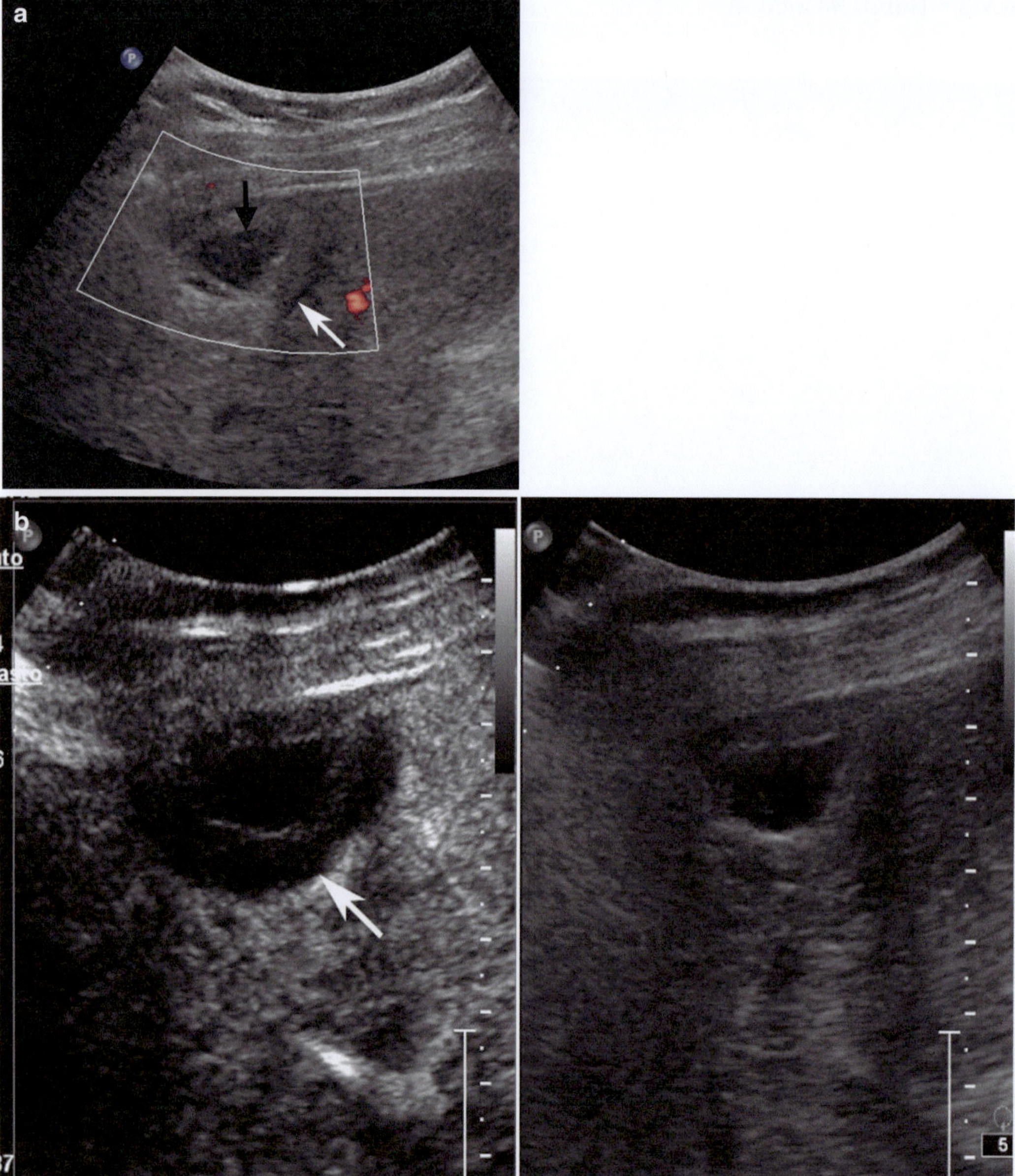

Fig. 6.9 Hepatocellular carcinoma treated with bipolar radiofrequency electrosurgical device in a 75-year-old man on 1 month follow-up. (**a**) Oblique ascending right subcostal baseline US image in a 57-year-old man reveals a 2 cm-sized isoechoic circumferential peripheral halo (*arrow*) surrounding a fluid collection (*black arrow*) at coagulated site in the subcapsular region in the V hepatic segment in absence of vascular signal at power-Doppler evaluation; (**b–d**) At CEUS, the lesion shows lack of contrast enhancement throughout the vascular study (*arrows*) as complete response

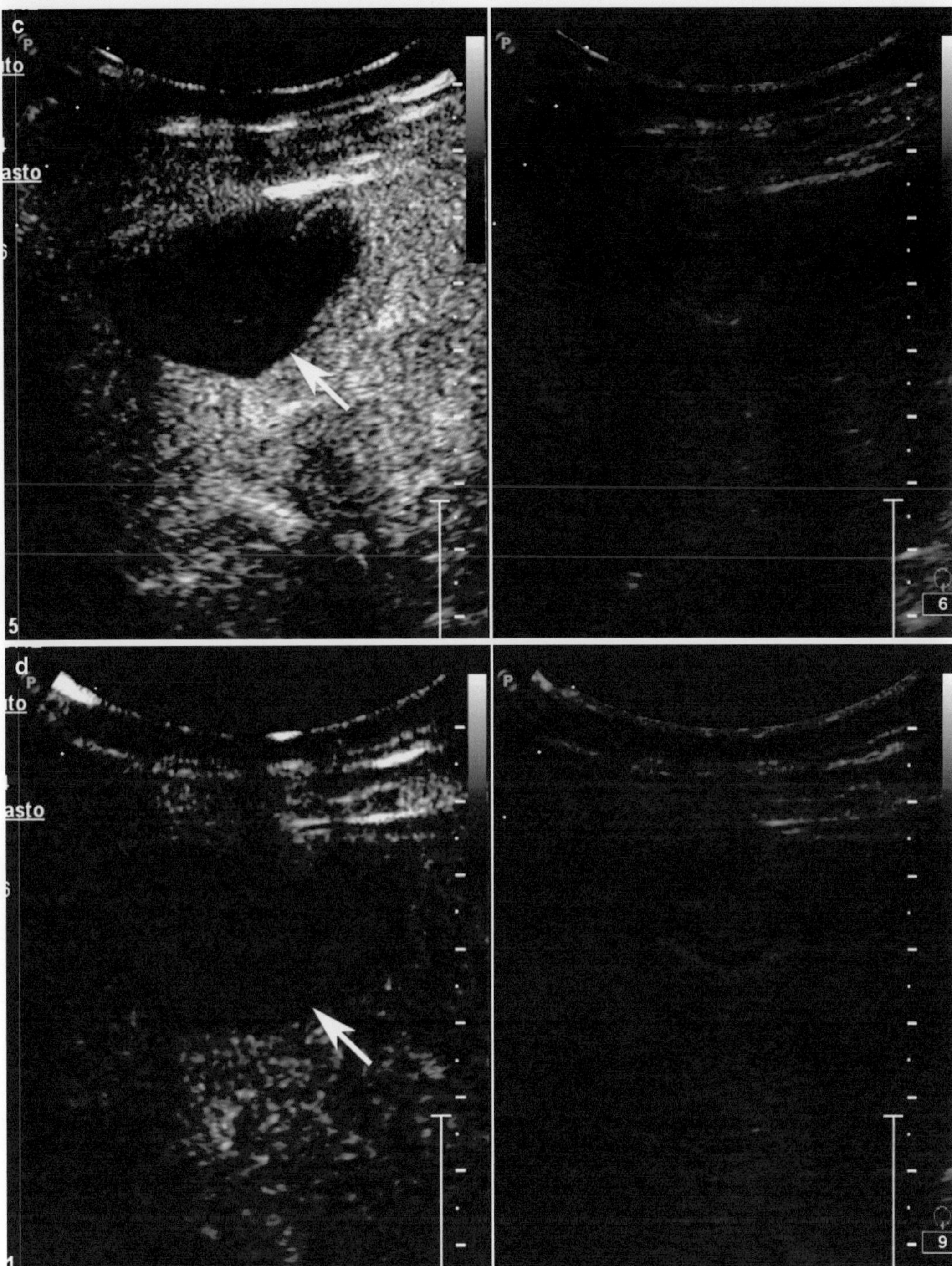

Fig. 6.9 (continued)

6.2   Systemic Treatment with Targeted Molecular Therapy

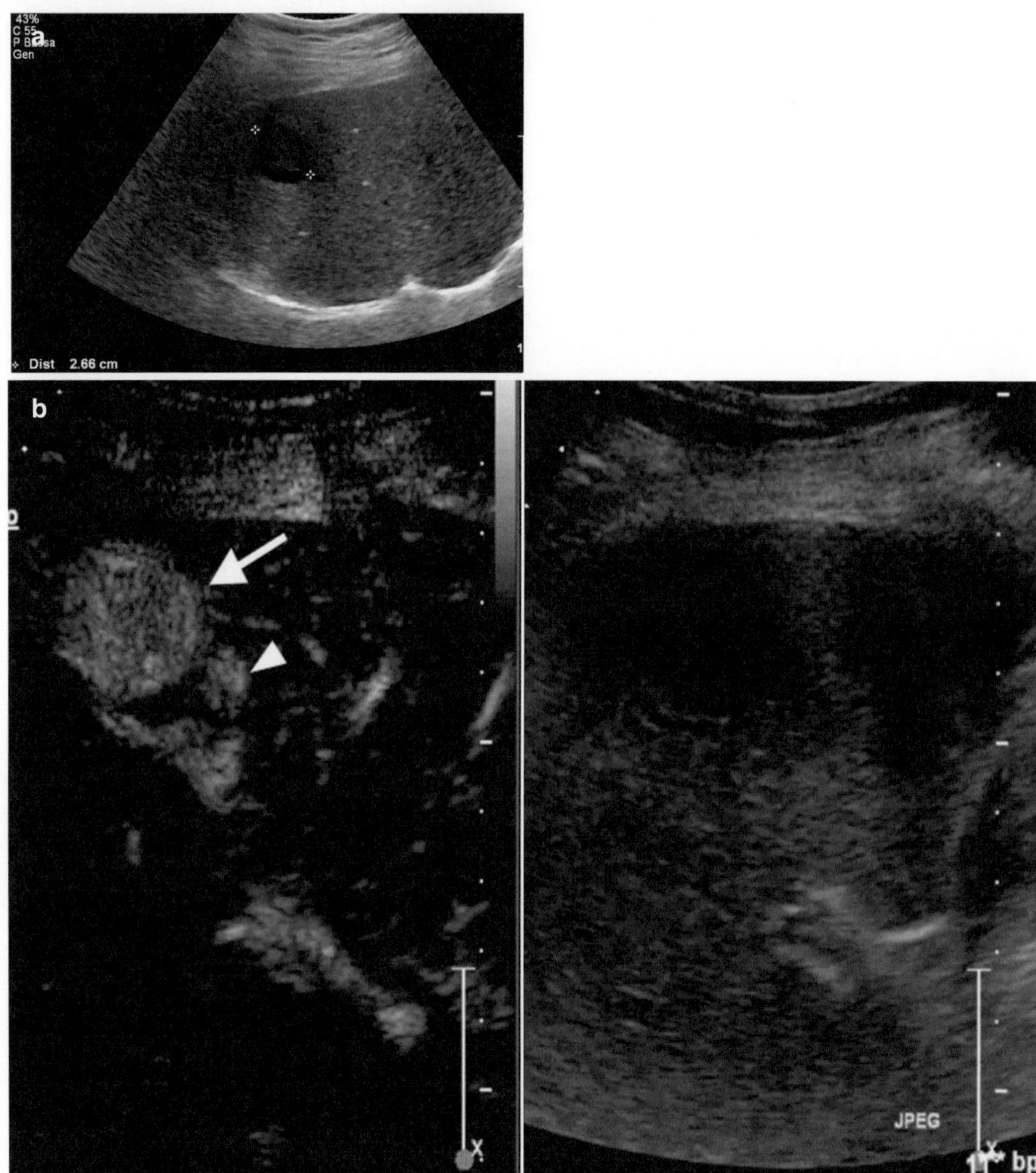

Fig. 6.10 Liver metastasis from GIST before and after treatment with antineoangiogenetic drug (Imatinib) in a 68-year-old woman. (**a**) Oblique ascending right subcostal baseline US image reveals a well-defined hypoechoic lesion sized 2.7 cm in the VII hepatic segment (calipers). (**b**) The lesion shows an intense and homogeneous contrast enhancement in the arterial phase (*arrow*). Nearby, another similar hypervascular lesion is evident (*arrowhead*). (**c**) After treatment, the first lesion is reduced in size on baseline US image (calipers). (**d**) At CEUS, it remains hypervascular (*arrow*), but the second one is no more evident

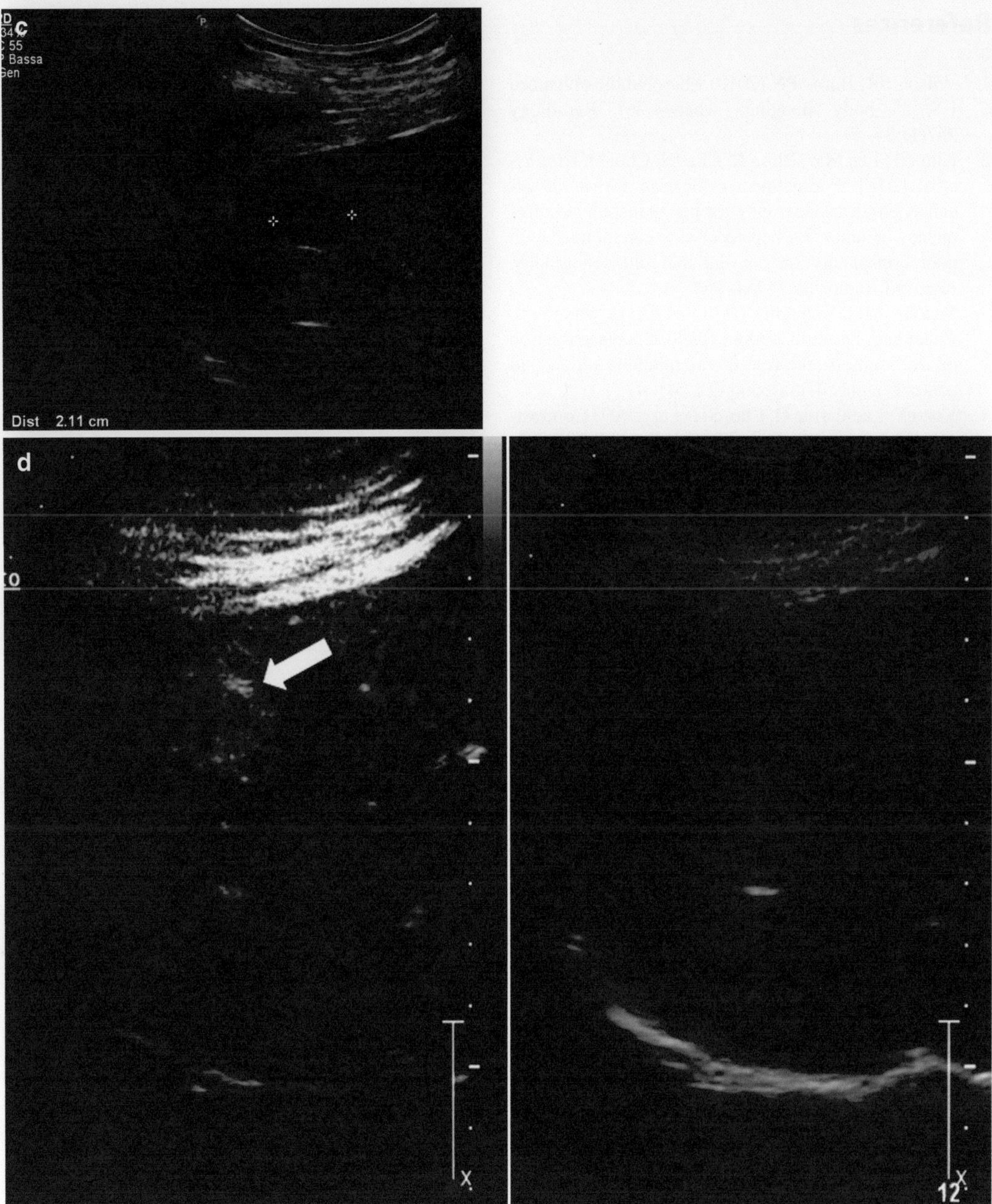

Fig. 6.10 (continued)

References

1. Wilson SR, Burns PN (2010) Microbubble-enhanced US in body imaging: what role? Radiology 257(1):24–39
2. Kim AY, Lee MW, Rhim H, Cha DI, Choi D, Kim YS et al (2013) Pretreatment evaluation with contrast-enhanced ultrasonography for percutaneous radiofrequency ablation of hepatocellular carcinomas with poor conspicuity on conventional ultrasonography. Korean J Radiol 14(5):754–763
3. Meloni MF, Livraghi T, Filice C, Lazzaroni S, Calliada F, Perretti L (2006) Radiofrequency ablation of liver tumors: the role of microbubble ultrasound contrast agents. Ultrasound Q 22:41–47
4. Kono Y, Lucidarme O, Choi SH et al (2007) Contrast-enhanced ultrasound as a predictor of treatment efficacy within 2 weeks after transarterial chemoembolization of hepatocellular carcinoma. J Vasc Interv Radiol 18:57–65
5. Solbiati L, Ierace T, Tonolini M, Cova L (2004) Guidance and monitoring of radiofrequency liver tumor ablation with contrast-enhanced ultrasound. Eur J Radiol 51:S19–S23
6. Morimoto M, Sugimori K, Shirato K (2002) Treatment of hepatocellular carcinoma with radiofrequency ablation: radiologic-histologic correlation during follow-up periods. Hepatology 460(35):1467–1475
7. Bartolotta TV, Taibbi A, Matranga D, Sandonato L, Asta S, Midiri M, Lagalla R (2012) Incidence of new foci of hepatocellular carcinoma after radiofrequency ablation: role of multidetector CT. Radiol Med 117(5):739–48. doi:10.1007/s11547-011-0752-z, Epub 2011 Nov 17. PubMed

As reported in the guidelines and good clinical practice recommendations for contrast-enhanced ultrasound (CEUS) in the liver, the use of CEUS is recommended for the following indications [1].

7.1 Focal Liver Lesions in the Noncirrhotic Liver

CEUS should be performed and interpreted with knowledge of the patient's clinical history and investigation findings. When the enhancement patterns are typical (in appropriate clinical settings), hemangiomas, focal nodular hyperplasia, focal fatty change, and malignancies can all be characterized with confidence. FLL with atypical enhancement patterns or studies that are technically suboptimal require further investigation mainly with CECT and/or CEMRI.

CEUS is indicated for lesion characterization in the following clinical situations:

- Incidental findings on routine ultrasound
- Lesion(s) or suspected lesion(s) detected with US in patients with a known history of a malignancy as an alternative to CT or MRI
- Need for a contrast study when CT and MRI contrasts are contraindicated
- Inconclusive MRI/CT
- Inconclusive cytology/histology results

Specificity and sensitivity are reduced in moderately or markedly fatty livers and with deeply positioned lesions.

7.2 Focal Liver Lesions in the Cirrhotic Liver

CEUS is recommended

- To characterize all nodules found on surveillance and routine US.
- To characterize nodules in cirrhosis and establish a diagnosis of HCC. It is a strong belief of the expert panel that CEUS is extremely useful, especially when performed immediately after nodule detection, to make a rapid diagnosis. However, CT or MRI are needed (unless contraindicated) to stage the disease before the treatment strategy is decided.
- Whether CEUS has a role as first-line investigation at the same level as CT or MRI is variably accepted in national and international guidelines. For example, CEUS is part of the Japanese guidelines on HCC [2, 3] but has been removed from the American guidelines [4]. This was partly justified by the fact that no UCA is licensed for the liver in the USA and additionally because of the risk of misdiagnosing CCC for HCC when CEUS is used alone (1–2 %). In practice, the likelihood of misdiagnosis is minimal when CEUS is performed by skilled operators [5].
- When CT or MRI is inconclusive, especially in nodules not suitable for biopsy
- To contribute to the selection of nodule(s) for biopsy when they are multiple or have different contrast patterns

© Springer International Publishing Switzerland 2015
T.V. Bartolotta et al., *Atlas of Contrast-enhanced Sonography of Focal Liver Lesions*,
DOI 10.1007/978-3-319-17539-3_7

- To monitor changes in size and enhancement patterns over time when a nodule is not diagnostic for HCC and is being followed
- After inconclusive histology

7.3   Detection of Metastatic Lesions

- To characterize indeterminate (usually small) lesions shown on either CECT or CEMRI
- To "rule out" liver metastases or abscesses unless conventional ultrasound shows typical findings
- For treatment planning in selected cases to assess the number and location of liver metastases either alone or as complementary to CECT and/or CEMRI
- Surveillance of oncology patients where CEUS has been useful previously, recommended to replace unenhanced US with CEUS for the evaluation of liver metastases in colorectal cancer after chemotherapy [6]

A potential pitfall is that small cysts, which were not seen on unenhanced US, are sometimes detected in late or postvascular phase scanning. Careful reevaluation with conventional US may help to show their cystic nature. In doubtful situations, a second contrast agent injection is recommended, looking for arterial phase enhancement, which indicates viable tumor tissue.

7.4   Monitoring Ablation Treatment

- As a complement to CECT and/or CEMRI for pretreatment staging and assessment of target lesion vascularity
- Facilitation of needle positioning in cases of incomplete or poor lesion delineation on unenhanced US
- Evaluation of the immediate treatment effect after ablation and guidance for immediate retreatment of residual unablated tumor.

Using this strategy, the rate of incomplete ablation in the first session is reported to decrease from 16 to 6 % [7]

- Assessment of local tumor progression when follow-up CECT or CEMRI are contraindicated or not conclusive. In addition to CECT and/or CEMRI, CEUS may be used in follow-up protocols

References

1. Claudon M, Dietrich CF, Choi BI, Cosgrove DO, Kudo M, Nolsøe CP, Piscaglia F, Wilson SR, Barr RG, Chammas MC, Chaubal NG, Chen MH, Clevert DA, Correas JM, Ding H, Forsberg F, Fowlkes JB, Gibson RN, Goldberg BB, Lassau N, Leen EL, Mattrey RF, Moriyasu F, Solbiati L, Weskott HP, Xu HX, World Federation for Ultrasound in Medicine (2013) European Federation of Societies for Ultrasound. Guidelines and good clinical practice recommendations for Contrast Enhanced Ultrasound (CEUS) in the liver – update 2012: a WFUMB-EFSUMB initiative incooperation with representatives of AFSUMB, AIUM, ASUM, FLAUS and ICUS. Ultrasound Med Biol 39(2):187–210. doi:10.1016/j.ultrasmedbio.2012.09.002
2. Kudo M, Okanoue T (2007) Management of hepatocellular carcinoma in Japan: consensus-based clinical practice manual proposed by the Japan Society of Hepatology. Oncology 72(Suppl 1):2–15
3. Kudo M, Izumi N, Kokudo N, Matsui O, Sakamoto M, Nakashima O, Kojiro M, Makuuchi M (2011) Management of hepatocellular carcinoma in Japan: Consensus-Based Clinical Practice Guidelines proposed by the Japan Society of Hepatology (JSH) 2010 updated version. Dig Dis 29:339–364
4. Bruix J, Sherman M (2011) Management of hepatocellular carcinoma: an update. Hepatology 53:1020–1022
5. Barreiros AP, Piscaglia F, Dietrich CF (2012) Contrast enhanced ultrasound for the diagnosis of hepatocellular carcinoma (HCC): comments on AASLD guidelines. J Hepatol 57(4):930–2. doi:10.1016/j.jhep.2012.04.018
6. Konopke R, Bunk A, Kersting S (2008) Contrast-enhanced ultrasonography in patients with colorectal liver metastases after chemotherapy. Ultraschall Med 29(Suppl 4):S203–S209
7. Chen MH, Yang W, Yan K, Zou MW, Solbiati L, Liu JB, Dai Y (2004) Large liver tumors: protocol for radiofrequency ablation and its clinical application in 110 patients–mathematic model, overlapping mode, and electrode placement process. Radiology 232:260–271